THE SCOUTING GUIDE TO WILDERNESS FIRST AID

MORE THAN 200 ESSENTIAL SKILLS FOR MEDICAL EMERGENCIES IN REMOTE ENVIRONMENTS

GRANT S. LIPMAN, MD, FACEP, FAWM

Clinical Associate Professor of Emergency Medicine

Director, Wilderness Medicine Section & Wilderness Medicine Fellowship

Stanford University School of Medicine

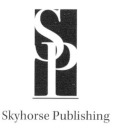

Skyhorse Publishing

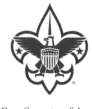

The Boy Scouts of America

This book is dedicated to Ashlie, Bennett, and Eva.
I look forward to sharing a lifetime of adventures with you.

Copyright © 2019 by Wildside Medical Education, LLC

Illustrations by Willie Azali and Rod Walinchus.

Printed under license from the Boy Scouts of America to Skyhorse
Publishing, Inc. For more information on the Boy Scouts of
America program, visit www.scouting.org.

Skyhorse Publishing books may be purchased in bulk at special
discounts for sales promotion, corporate gifts, fund-raising, or
educational purposes. Special editions can also be created to
specifications. For details, contact the Special Sales Department,
Skyhorse Publishing, 307 West 36th Street, 11th Floor, New York,
NY 10018 or info@skyhorsepublishing.com.

Skyhorse® and Skyhorse Publishing® are registered trademarks of
Skyhorse Publishing, Inc.®, a Delaware corporation.

Visit our website at www.skyhorsepublishing.com.

10 9 8 7 6 5 4 3 2 1

Library of Congress Cataloging-in-Publication Data available on
file.

Cover design by Brian Peterson

Print ISBN: 978-1-5107-3971-0
Ebook ISBN: 978-1-5107-3973-4

Printed in China

DISCLAIMER

It is the responsibility of the reader to take a wilderness first aid or equivalent training course, as the information contained in this book is not intended as a substitution for a course or practical experience. To the fullest extent of the law, neither the Author nor the Publisher assumes any liability for any injury, disability, death, and/or damage to persons or property resulting from any use or operation of any methods, products, instructions, or ideas contained in the material herein.

TABLE OF CONTENTS

✚

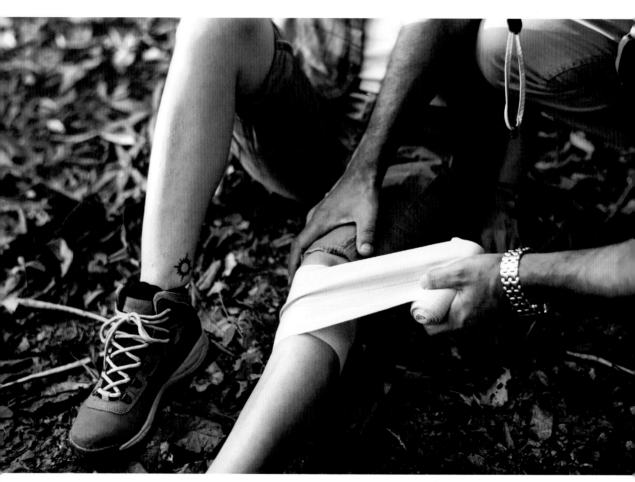

An in-depth knowledge of wilderness first aid can come in handy.

INTRODUCTION

Five years ago I published the *Wilderness First Aid Handbook*. That book was the culmination of several years of discussions with students, instructors, and educators while serving as Medical Advisor for Stanford Outdoor Education. I had wanted to provide protocols that could deliver logical and useful guidance for first responders whose depth of medical knowledge was a sixteen-hour wilderness first aid (WFA) course. I attempted to stay within the bounds of the curriculum and course that have been adopted and taught throughout the United States. In preparation for this Scouting edition, I revisited the doctrine and the evidence that forms the backbone of wilderness first aid,

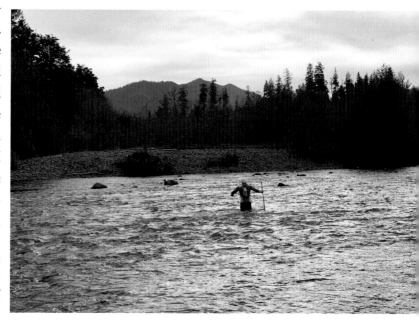

Before going on a trip in the wilderness, consider taking a first-aid course. *Credit: Grant Lipman*

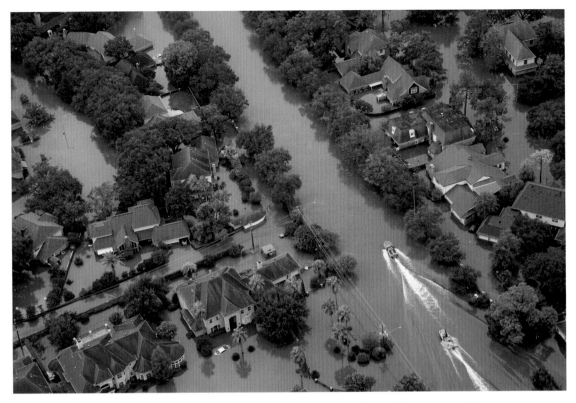

Wilderness first aid skills may come in handy in areas affected by natural disasters.

and remembered the lessons (delivered and received) over the years from my emergency medicine residents and wilderness medicine fellows in the Stanford Department of Emergency Medicine. I decided to expand the scope of this edition to reflect both the WFA core curriculum as well as complex concepts and skills, as often readers have a thirst for advanced knowledge.

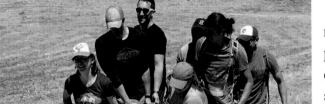

Wilderness first aid is the assessment and treatment of an ill or injured person in an environment where definitive medical care by a professional or rapid transport to definitive care is unavailable. People who work,

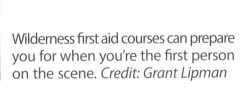

Wilderness first aid courses can prepare you for when you're the first person on the scene. *Credit: Grant Lipman*

 SCOUTING GUIDE TO WILDERNESS FIRST AID

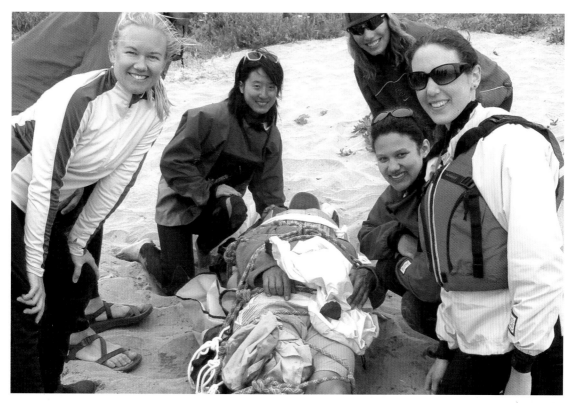

Wilderness first aid courses can teach you how to assess an ill or injured individual.
Credit: Grant Lipman

live, travel, and recreate in the outdoors have specialized medical needs not adequately fulfilled by traditional first aid. Wilderness first aid fills this gap. Remote locations, arduous conditions, paucity of diagnostic and therapeutic equipment, and a need to make critical decisions, often without outside communication, define wilderness medicine as a specialty. These conditions may be

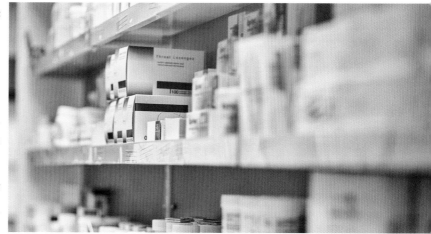

You can purchase most of the medicines in this book over the counter.

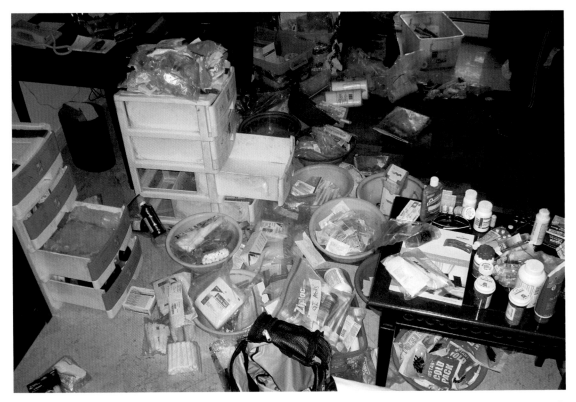

Consult with a doctor about any medicines you carry or prescriptions you may need.
Credit: Grant Lipman

found in remote wilderness, the developing world, or even in wealthy urban areas beset by natural disasters. This book is to be used as a guide to augment the skills and training learned in a typical wilderness first aid course. The intention is to assist the lay public, outdoor professionals, and instructors as well as members of wilderness first aid classes with useful and practical information that complements their training. Some elective skills are included, which the individual can decide to include depending on his or her comfort level and specific training.

This book is written for those who have basic first aid knowledge, not necessarily those with advanced degrees in medicine or pre-hospital care. The American Heart Association has limited components of its resuscitation curriculum, recognizing that some tasks may be difficult for laypersons to competently perform. Similarly, this book acknowledges that certain knowledge and procedures are outside the scope of the average wilderness first aid provider's knowledge, and thus strives to limit the use of technical terms or advanced techniques that may be unfamiliar to some readers or impractical based on the wilderness setting.

✚ SCOUTING GUIDE TO WILDERNESS FIRST AID

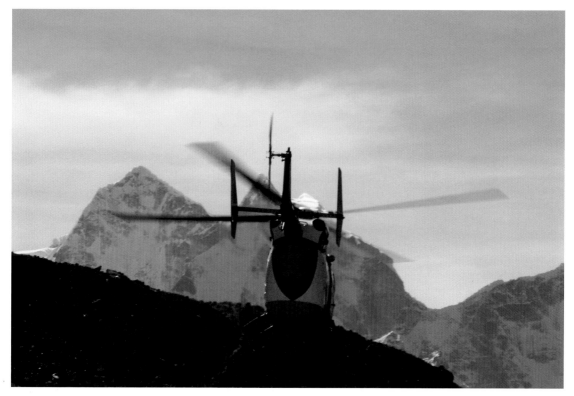

Depending on where you are in the wilderness during an emergency, medical personnel may need a boat or helicopter to reach you. *Credit: Grant Lipman*

This book provides easy-to-follow protocols and instructions to assist those encountering most wilderness emergencies.

While the contents of this book are meant to assist in managing a medical emergency in a remote environment, the information is applicable to any setting where the reader is first on the scene. The protocols contained in this book are to be used as guidelines and are by no means a substitution for common sense or definitive medical care. A rescuer is liable for his or her own actions and should never undertake a medical procedure he or she feels uncomfortable with or which is not absolutely necessary unless the rescuer believes the victim may lose their life or limb without intervention.

Most medicines discussed in this book can be purchased over the counter. Consult with a doctor concerning the potential side effects, complications, or contraindications of any medications you carry. Similarly, ensure that there are no known allergies to the medicines you use.

Travel in the wilderness is an inherently risky activity, as one often travels to remote locations for the adventure, solitude, and serenity provided. Ultimately, the ethos of self-reliance found in the backcountry is epitomized by a wilderness medical emergency. These protocols assume knowledge and implementation of patient assessment systems that should not be ignored when acting on these protocols. Familiarize yourself with the information within these pages before venturing into the backcountry to minimize the chances that an accident will have to be an emergency.

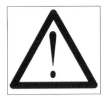

This danger symbol next to the "red flags" of a patient's symptoms serves as an indicator of a dangerous disease process that may necessitate imminent evacuation to definitive medical care. If any of these "red flags" are observed, start early preparations for a potential evacuation. Consideration of the terrain, time of day, and weather are all potential issues in expediting a timely evacuation.

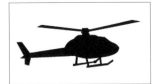

This helicopter symbol next to the "evacuate" assumes a medical emergency that requires a higher level of care via Emergency Medical Services (EMS). All evacuations assume the emergency is taking place in a setting where communication is likely not possible. The severity of the emergency, the potential for the patient to decompensate, the availability (or lack thereof) of outside communication, and the logistical and timely constraints of a rescue versus self-evacuation all need to be taken into consideration. **If patients are able to ambulate on their own without endangering themselves or others, self-evacuation may be a quicker and better option in the wilderness environment.** If a victim is unable to walk, or you expect that the ability to ambulate may shortly become compromised, you should likely send for a rescue. If the decision is made to send a messenger to initiate an EMS rescue, two people (buddy system) are better than one to ensure the safe delivery of both the message and messengers.

> If the reader of this book is unsure of the necessity of an evacuation, they should likely err on the side of caution. "When in doubt, get out."

CHAPTER 1

ASSESSMENT SYSTEM/CPR

Before you are able to administer first aid, an assessment must be made in an orderly process to ensure that both the rescuer and the patient are kept safe. Providing aid for a traumatic injury is similar to considering the causes of a sickness or random pains. The processes are the same, and a systematic approach to the problem will allow a logical step-by-step assessment, stabilization, and treatment. In the setting of trauma, rushing to provide care without

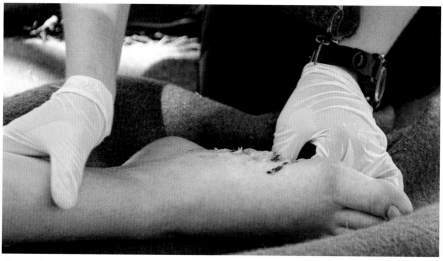

If you have gloves on the scene of the emergency, use them to protect both you and the patient.

an orderly assessment of the scene may inadvertently turn the rescuer into a victim. Keep in mind the adage, "Don't just stand there, do something." The initial assessment should consider hazards that could cause immediate injuries to the people attempting to assist the injured person.

Scene Size-Up

- Ensure it is safe for the rescuer to approach the patient.
- Consider the number of patients.
- Consider the mechanism of injury (MOI), or how the patient may have been injured and the need for immediate spine immobilization (*see* Trauma).
- If body substances are present, consider gloves or eye protection precaution in order to protect both you and the patient.

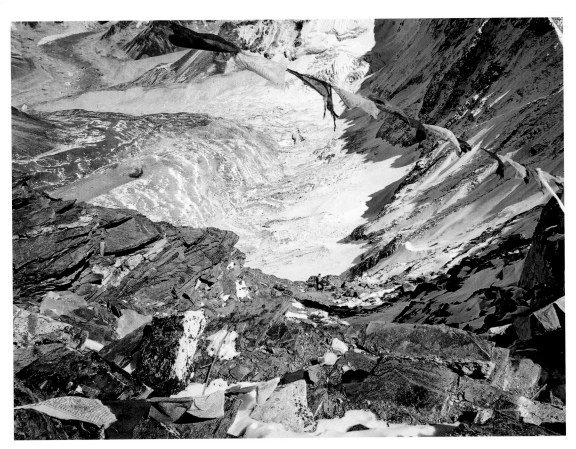

Ensure the scene is safe for the rescuer prior to approaching a potential patient.
Credit: Grant Lipman

SCOUTING GUIDE TO WILDERNESS FIRST AID

Primary Assessment

After the scene has been assessed and you are certain it is safe to approach the patient, the next step is to identify immediate threats to life. If a problem is found, stop and fix it before moving on. The primary assessment should identify potential causes of death, including lack of oxygen from a blocked airway or inadequate breathing, loss of circulation from bleeding (either internal or external) or inadequate pumping from the heart, damage to the brain or spinal cord, or extremes of the environment or metabolism. If there is a patient who has a decreased level of responsiveness (LOR) and cannot respond, you may need to use your CPR training. If multiple victims are encountered, assessing the entire scene and determining where you can do the most good to the most people should dictate your priority. For example, you may need to apply a tourniquet to a heavily bleeding limb before you check the breathing on a non-responsive person.

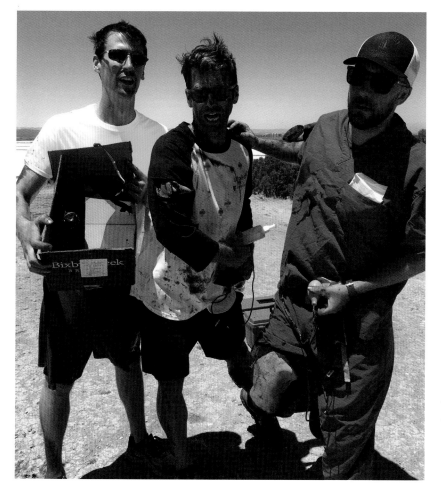

It may be necessary to control the bleeding to an injured limb prior to checking the breathing. *Credit: Grant Lipman*

Primary Assessment Procedure

- Introduce and identify yourself as you approach the patient.
- Obtain verbal consent to treat them.
- Establish responsiveness.
- Level of responsiveness (LOR): A-V-P-U—Alert, Verbal, Pain, Unresponsive.

ABCDE

- **A**irway
  - ➢ Check the patient's airway.
  - ➢ If a patient can talk, he or she has an open airway.
  - ➢ If necessary, open the airway by the head tilt/chin lift.

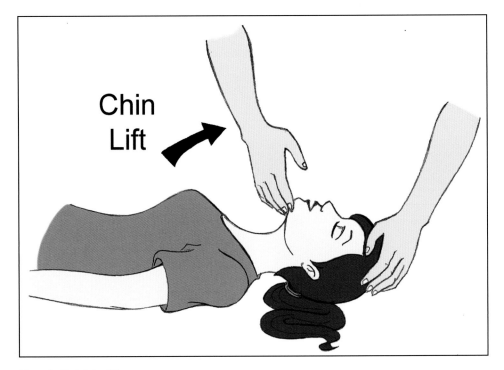

Head tilt/chin lift.

  - ➢ Look in the mouth to clear any obstructions.
  - ➢ Heimlich maneuver/abdominal thrusts if the person appears to be choking or if there is an obstructing foreign body.

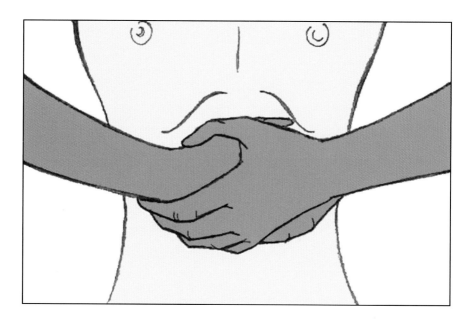

Hands position for Heimlich maneuver.

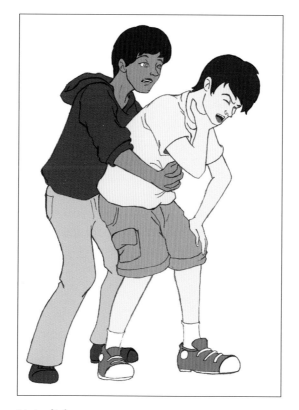

Heimlich maneuver.

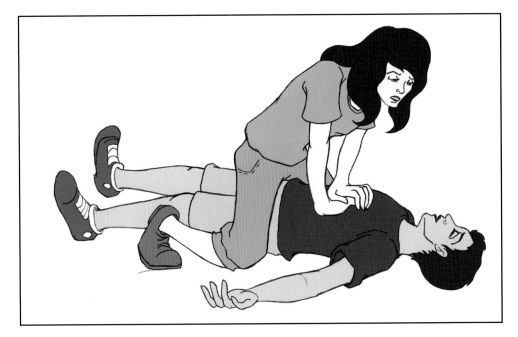

Abdominal thrusts for an unconscious choking victim.

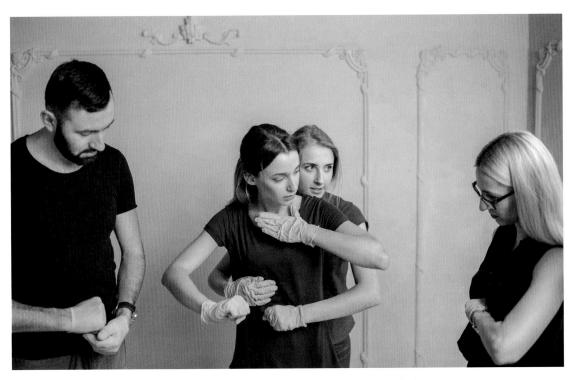

First aid courses can teach you how to properly give the Heimlich maneuver.

  SCOUTING GUIDE TO WILDERNESS FIRST AID

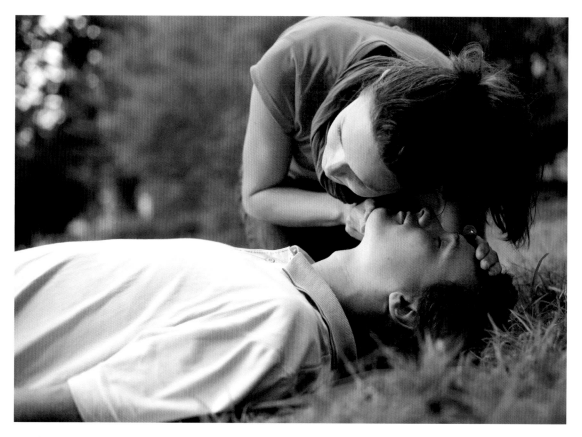

Look and listen to see if the patient is breathing. If they aren't, proceed to CPR.

- **B**reathing
  - ➤ Look and listen for breathing.
  - ➤ No breathing? (*see* CPR).
  - ➤ Assess if the breathing is difficult or painful (*see* Chest Pain, Chest Trauma, and/or Lung Problems).
- **C**irculation
  - ➤ Check to see if there is obvious major bleeding.
  - ➤ If massive bleeding or rapid pulse, check for site of bleeding and take appropriate action through either direct pressure or application of a tourniquet (*see* Wound Care).
  - ➤ Feel for a pulse.
  - ➤ No pulse? (*see* CPR)

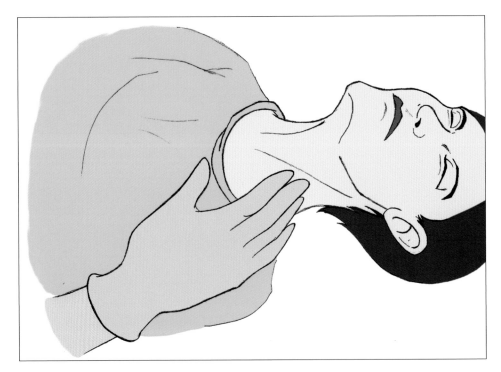

Feeling for a pulse.

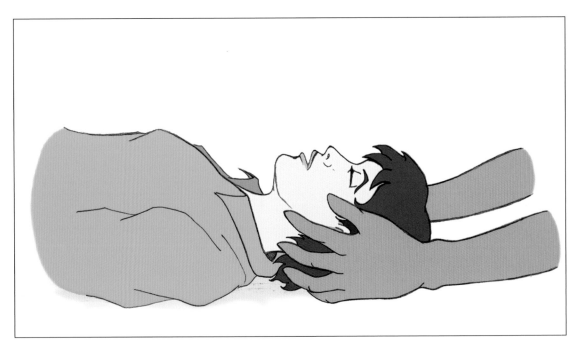

Spinal immobilization.

- **D**ecide/**D**isability
  - ➤ Consider the MOI and decide early if there is a necessity for spinal immobilization and control the head (*see* Trauma).
- **E**xposure/**E**nvironment
  - ➤ Expose serious wounds for full evaluation and treatment. Consider environmental causes (heat, cold, lightning) for the injury or illness as well as protecting the patient from further environmental stressors as treatment progresses (i.e., place on an insulating pad sooner rather than later in the care).

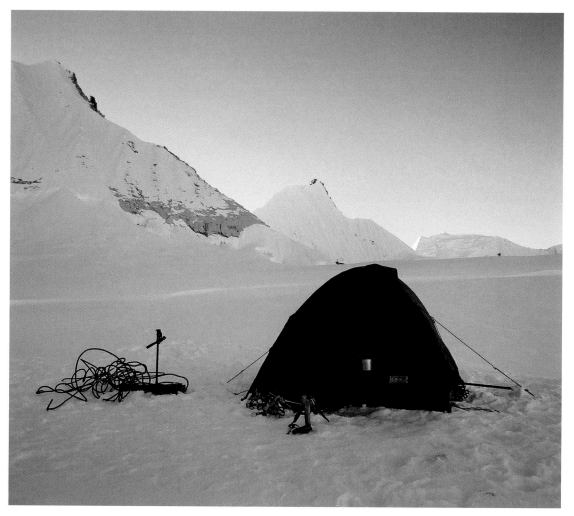

Consider possible environmental causes, such as cold temperature, for the patient's injury.
Credit: Grant Lipman

Secondary Assessment

Once evaluation of any immediate life-threatening events is complete, you are ready to perform a comprehensive and focused assessment of the injury and illness. This will involve gathering a complete history and performing a thorough physical exam from head to toe in a systematic manner. The initial survey should have found and corrected immediate critical conditions; the secondary assessment will now determine if other less obvious injuries can be identified. For example, a broken bone is painful and may be a distraction to both the patient and rescuer, but may make a rescuer overlook other more serious injuries.

The secondary assessment should be thorough, with direct and simple questions. Pushing everywhere may elicit subtle areas of tenderness. Sliding a hand under a shirt may find a hidden area of blood loss. The outcome of this secondary assessment will lead to system specific protocols and decisions for treatment and/or evacuation to definitive medical care. Most methodologic approaches start at the head and work down towards the feet. Always let the patient know what you are doing and where you are about to touch so they are not alarmed or offended. While performing the secondary survey, move the patient as little as possible to avoid aggravating any injuries.

Secondary Assessment Procedure

- Determine the chief complaint (what hurts or is bothering the patient).
- History of the illness (when and how it happened).
- **SAMPLE** History:
  - ➤ Symptoms.
  - ➤ Allergies (to medications/latex).
  - ➤ Medications.
  - ➤ Pertinent medical history.
  - ➤ Last food or drink.
  - ➤ Events that happened which may be relevant to the chief complaint.
- Check vital signs: heart rate, respiratory rate.

Physical Exam

Ask the patient where it hurts, and then, when feeling gently, ask if it hurts to be touched there. You may need to remove clothing to completely visualize the injury.

- Head. Feel the skull for swelling and depressions, look for drainage from the ears, nose, and mouth. Have the patient feel their teeth to ensure they match up, and can open and close their jaw naturally and without pain.

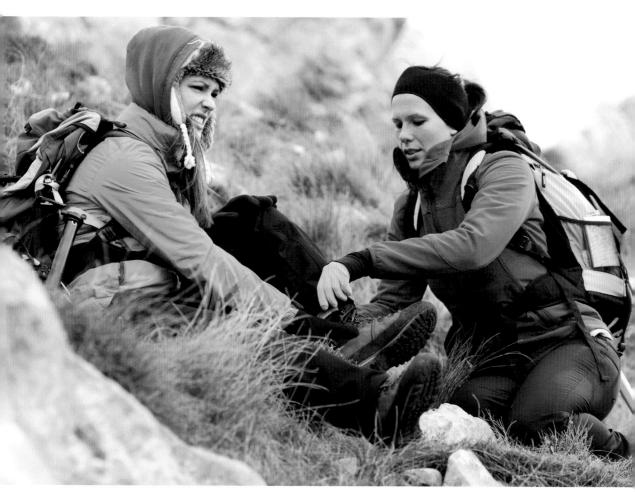

A physical exam will help you get a better idea of how to treat the patient's injury.

- Neck. Differentiate midline spinal tenderness from non-midline tense muscles and tenderness.
- Chest. Press on both sides of the chest, listen, and feel for abnormal sounds.
- Abdomen. Press on all quadrants to differentiate pain from tenderness.
- Pelvis. Gently push on the bony prominences of the pelvis at the hips.
- Legs. Feel and look for symmetry and full range of movement.
- Arms. Feel and look for symmetry and full range of movement. Press on one arm at a time, and be sure to check wrists, hands, and fingers.
- Back. Press on every bone from the top to the bottom of the spine. Consider log-roll precautions if you suspect a spinal injury.

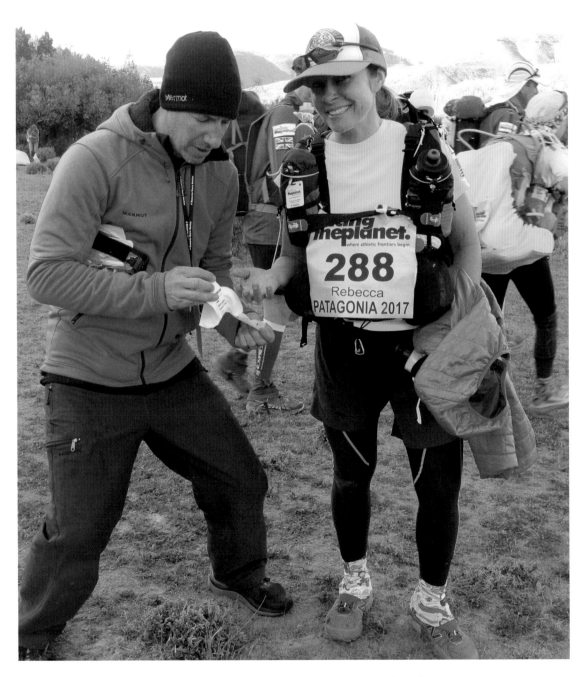

After helping your patient, make sure to document as much information as you can as soon as possible. *Credit: Grant Lipman*

The SOAP Note

Collect information and write it down as soon as possible. Document what you do and any changes to the patient. This is important for both patient care and to protect the first-aid responder. If the patient requires evacuation, the SOAP note will allow for a continuation of care and concise communication of the events that transpired in the pre-hospital setting.

- **S**ubjective/**S**ummary of the patient's age, complaints, and occurrences.
- **O**bjective/**O**bservations of the patient, vital signs, and SAMPLE history.
- **A**ssessments of what you think is wrong, and assess any changes to the patient and what may develop or change.
- **P**lan what you are going to do, and whether the patient needs an intervention or evacuation.

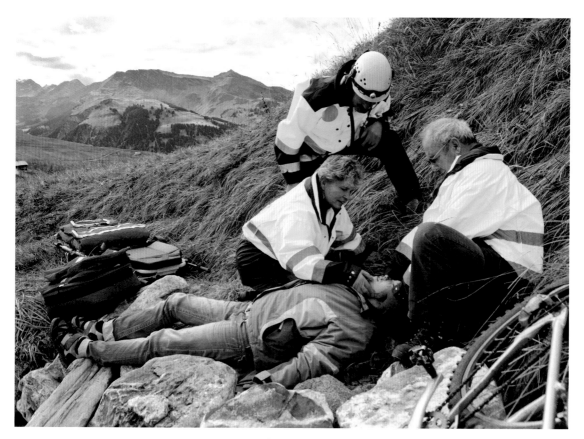

After evaluating the patient, determine whether or not they need an evacuation.

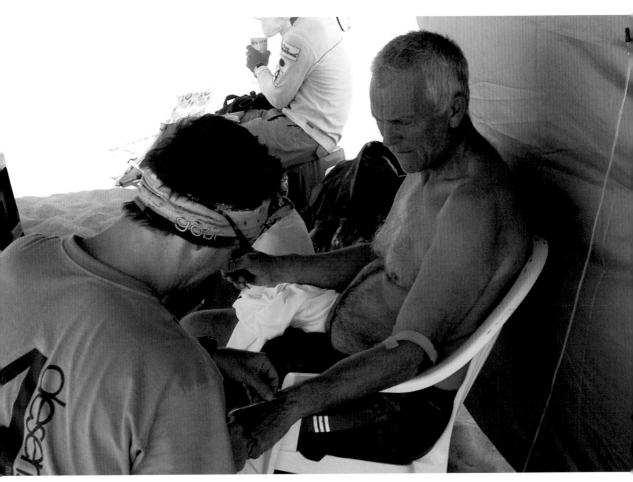

A careful history and physical can help determine the cause of abdominal pain.
Credit: Grant Lipman

CHAPTER 2

ABDOMINAL PAIN

Abdominal pain is a potentially concerning although not uncommon complaint. Even in a hospital with all the resources of a laboratory, ultrasounds, and CT scans it can still be a challenging diagnosis. In a wilderness setting with no tools other than a thorough history and physical exam, care must be taken in evaluating the patient for clues that may necessitate an evacuation for a problem that may require medical or surgical intervention. While this is a challenging diagnostic problem in the backcountry, a thorough patient interview will be of great assistance in differentiating the causes. Abdominal pain can range from mild discomfort to a serious or deadly event. When performing the secondary assessment, press gently on all quadrants of the stomach with a flat open palm. The pain and exam may change over time. Pay attention for red flags and have a low index of suspicion to evacuate if symptoms progress or pain that lasts more than twenty-four hours.

Pain in the right upper quadrant of the abdomen may be from a problem with the gallbladder. Gallbladder disease is more common in overweight people over forty, also in women. The pain may initially be episodic, with an onset after eating, but may become constant and severe. There is no burning or "sour stomach" associated with gallbladder pain. If a fever is present this may represent an infected gallbladder, which is a surgical emergency and necessitates intravenous antibiotics and evacuation.

Pain in the right lower quadrant raises the possibility of appendicitis. This can occur in any age range. The pain typically starts arounds the belly button and then the discomfort

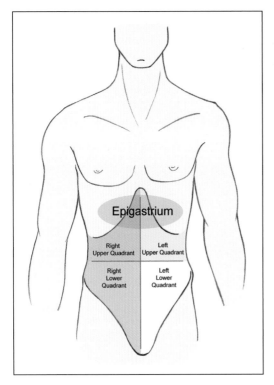

Abdomen schematic.

migrates to the right lower quadrant, halfway between the belly button and top of the right hip bone. Ask questions specifically to elicit when and where the pain started, and where it is now. The localization of pain and tenderness to the right lower quadrant should raise the suspicion of acute appendicitis. It may present with diarrhea and/or vomiting. Presence of this pain with a fever, increased pain with movement or pushing on other areas of the abdomen all should raise concern for a surgical emergency and evacuation. However, if someone with abdominal pain can walk comfortably and jump up and down with no discomfort, this should be reassuring that it is less likely acute appendicitis.

Left lower quadrant abdominal pain can be from diverticulitis, an infection of small outpouchings of the large bowel. This is more common in the middle-aged and elderly, and usually presents with constant, dull, and worsening pain. It can present with diarrhea, but unlike the crampy abdominal pain often found with diarrhea, this pain is localized to the left lower quadrant and reproducible with palpation. As this infection progresses, a fever usually occurs and evacuation to a hospital is needed with intravenous antibiotics and sometimes even surgery.

Diarrhea is the passage of loose or watery stools. It can be very common on trips, especially when there is poor hygiene. The watery bowel movements may present with crampy abdominal pain, sweats, malaise and fatigue, exhaustion, nausea and/or vomiting, and fevers and chills. The diarrhea can range from a mild nuisance to total debilitation. If proper hygiene is not maintained, diarrhea can easily spread through a camp, affecting lots of people. Most diarrhea while traveling is caused by ingested bacteria, and can be prevented by hand washing and water treatment. Water should be boiled, treated, or filtered before ingesting. Food should be peeled and hands washed or sanitized before eating and after having a bowel movement. Diarrhea may be caused by viruses, which are notorious for spreading among members of an outing, and while self-limited, may make life miserable for several days. Proper latrine placement (at least two hundred meters from camp) and having a "no shoes in tent" policy can minimize the risk of spreading diarrhea-causing organisms.

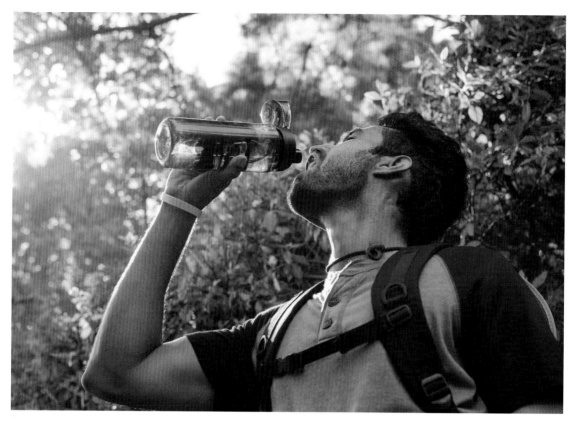
Hydrating can assist with preventing constipation.

Symptoms: Constipation (No Stool for Several Days)
- Hard stools, bloating, distention.
- Crampy, intermittent, generalized (four quadrant) pain.
- Pain may be greater in the left lower quadrant of the abdomen.
- Patient may be doubled-over in distress.

Caffeinated drinks like coffee or tea can stimulate the bowels and lessen abdominal pain from constipation.

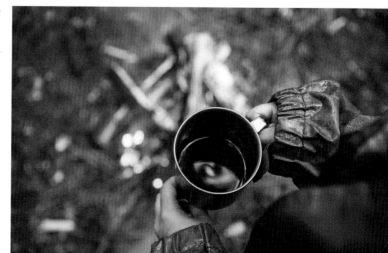

⚠️ **Red Flags:** Presence of vomiting or fever with constipation, history of small bowel obstruction, or history of abdominal surgery.

Treatment
- Maintain hydration with clear fluids.
- If dehydrated, rehydrate with electrolyte-containing fluids.
- Give caffeinated drinks (coffee, tea, hot chocolate) to stimulate the bowels.
- Give fiber or sips of mineral oil (if available).
- Give laxative (if available).
- Offer adequate latrine time.

Symptoms: Nausea, Vomiting, Diarrhea
- Crampy or sharp intermittent pain.
- Possibly associated with fever and/or fatigue.
- Diarrhea may be loose, watery, or with mucus.

⚠️ **Red Flags:** Diarrhea with blood, fever, or vomiting with blood.

Treatment
- Control the nausea with sips of herbal tea and Pepcid as needed (as directed by the instruction label).
- Rehydrate with electrolyte-containing solution. Start slowly (sips every five minutes), then when tolerating liquids, rehydrate until urine is clear.
- Ibuprofen or Tylenol as needed for pain (as directed by instruction label).
- If mild diarrhea (four to six stools/day), can treat with Pepto-Bismol (as directed by instruction label).
- If frequent diarrhea (six or more stools/day but no fever or blood in stool), treat with Imodium (as directed by instruction label).

Symptoms: Lower Abdominal Pain in a Female
- May be a dull or sharp pain, constant or intermittent, and may be one sided.
- May include vaginal bleeding.

⚠️ **Red Flags:** History of missed or irregular menstrual period, atypical from regular menstrual pain, one-sided pain.

Treatment

- Ibuprofen (as directed by instruction label).
- Pregnancy test.

Symptoms: Epigastric Pain or "Sour Stomach"

- Pain at the top of the abdomen, may be burning, radiating up into chest or neck.
- Eating food or lying flat may worsen pain. Intermittent generalized cramping is common.

⚠ **Red Flags:** Black tarry stools, bloody stools, fever, history of peptic ulcer disease, or history of heart disease.

Treatment

- Pepcid or Pepto-Bismol (as directed by instruction label).
- Hydrate.
- Cold water.

Symptoms: Trauma (Blunt or Penetrating)

- Mild pain.
- Nausea.
- Pain worsened by flexing abdominal wall muscles.

⚠ **Red Flags:** Any hole in the skin or protruding bowel, pain that is progressively becoming more severe, pain worsened with any movement or palpation, pain in the shoulders after abdominal injury, bloating or persistent vomiting, fever, or any dizziness, rapid breathing, rapid pulse, or altered level of responsiveness. Evacuate any penetrating abdominal trauma.

Treatment

- Sips of cold water.
- Tylenol for pain.
- Protruding bowel covered with clean moist (sterile) gauze, with several dry layers of gauze affixed on top..
- Leave penetrating object in place and stabilized (*see* Wound Care).
- Have a low threshold for immediate evacuation with significant blunt abdominal trauma.

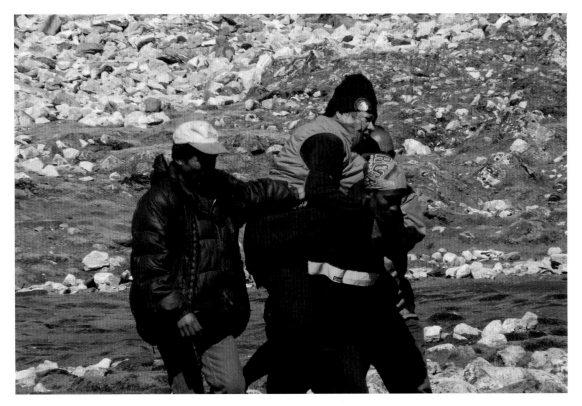

Sometimes abdominal pain can be a sign that surgical intervention is necessary. In this case, it is important to evacuate the patient. *Credit: Grant Lipman*

 Evacuate: Any patient with abdominal pain who also has:
- Abdominal pain worsened with movement.
- Persistent localized pain for more than twelve hours.
- Intermittent diffuse pain lasting more than twenty-four hours.
- Black tarry stools.
- Fevers for eight hours with abdominal pain.
- Blood in vomit, stool, or urine (other than flecks of blood).
- Positive pregnancy test with abdominal pain.
- Inability to tolerate fluids.
- Combination of: sunken eyes, dry lining of the mouth, decreased urine output, and/ or generalized weakness, dizziness.
- Any penetrating trauma.
- Blunt trauma with red flags.

  SCOUTING GUIDE TO WILDERNESS FIRST AID

CHAPTER 3

ALLERGIC REACTION AND ANAPHYLAXIS

An allergic reaction can be set off by a bug bite, contact with a plant, or a food allergy. Symptoms of an allergic reaction range from mild to severe, the most severe of which is a life-threatening emergency called anaphylaxis. Most anaphylaxis will occur within one hour of onset of symptoms. People who develop anaphylaxis usually present with an allergic reaction initially that progresses. However, anaphylaxis can present abruptly as an isolated and catastrophic event. Allergic reactions can reoccur (rebound), so it is imperative to continue the entire course of treatment. Any patient who is suspected of having or is being treated for anaphylaxis should be immediately evacuated. Epinephrine is reserved for cases of severe allergic reaction and/or anaphylaxis; this is a potent prescription drug that can be dan-

Insect bites or stings can cause allergic reactions.

gerous to both provider and recipient if used incorrectly. Administrators need to be trained in the unique delivery of the drug.

Symptoms

- **Mild (may be diffuse):** Red or blotchy skin, raised welts, itching, burning, red or watery eyes.
- **Moderate:** Skin rash and swelling to face or over entire body, sense of throat scratchiness or fullness, abdominal pain.
- **Severe/Anaphylaxis:** Shortness of breath, wheezing when breathing, tongue/lip swelling, inability to speak or only few word sentences, difficulty swallowing, and/or altered level of responsiveness.

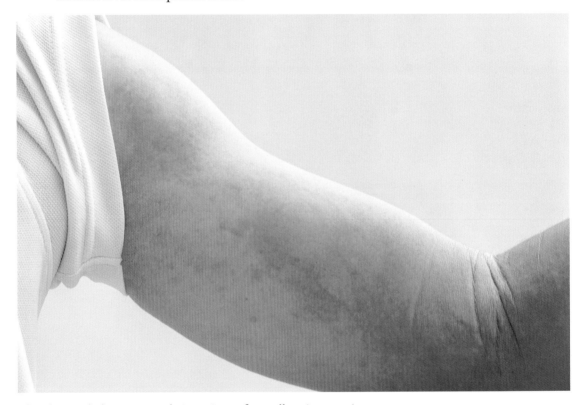

Blotchy, red skin or a rash is a sign of an allergic reaction.

⚠ **Red Flags:** Any symptom of moderate or severe allergic reaction or anaphylaxis.

Treatment

- Remove the offending allergen from the patient or the patient from the perceived offending trigger or environment.
- If a localized reaction, apply corticosteroid cream.
- **Mild and Moderate:** Benadryl and Pepcid (as directed by instruction label) for three days.
- **Severe/Anaphylaxis: <u>EpiPen instructions:</u>** 1) Pull off the safety cap. 2) Hold the EpiPen by grasping the shaft and placing the tip of the unit against the outer thigh, halfway between the hip and knee (ideally against the skin, but can be used through thin clothing). 3) Push the unit against the thigh until it clicks, which releases the hidden needle and delivery of medication. 4) Hold in place for a count of ten. May repeat in five to fifteen minutes if initial dose is ineffective or symptoms recur. Add all Mild and Moderate allergic reaction medicines.

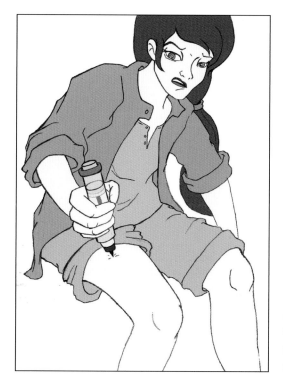

An EpiPen is an effective way to treat a severe allergic reaction or anaphylaxis.

Evacuate: Any patient who has received epinephrine. Any allergic reaction that does not improve with optimum treatment. Continue medications during evacuation.

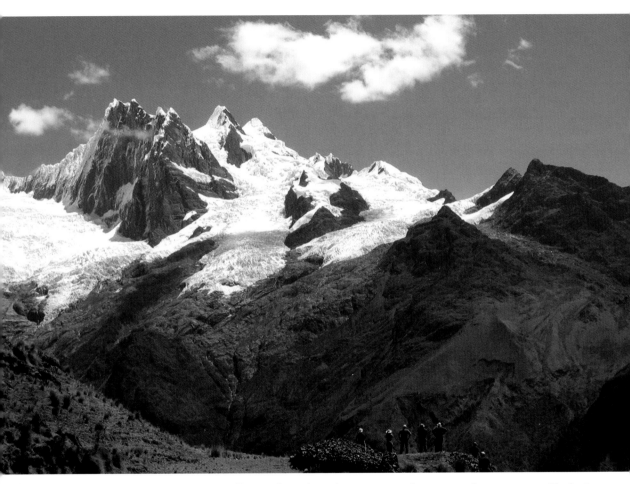

When traveling rapidly to altitudes above 8,000 feet, people are more likely to experience altitude illness. *Credit: Grant Lipman*

CHAPTER 4
ALTITUDE ILLNESS

Altitude illness results from the body's inability to adjust to the relatively low ambient oxygen concentration in the atmosphere at high altitudes. The amount of oxygen in the air stays a relatively constant 21 percent, but as altitude is gained, the amount of oxygen in the air decreases with lowered barometric pressures. So there is less inhaled oxygen the higher one ascends. For example, at 19,000 feet (5,757 meters) there is half the barometric pressure as sea level, so about half the available oxygen per breath. The compensatory response of the body upon ascending to high altitude to optimize the delivery of oxygen to the tissues is called acclimatization. Acclimatization is best accomplished by a gradual graded ascent with rest days. For example, while someone in a hot air balloon who rapidly ascended to the height of Mount Everest (with 28 percent of the oxygen of sea level) would rapidly pass out and then die, people have successfully climbed the mountain without oxygen, because they acclimatized. A gradual ascent will maximize the chances for the body to successfully handle the stress of a relatively low oxygen environment, and allow one to feel well.

The body's normal response to high altitude includes an increased breathing rate to deliver the amount of oxygen to your body; increased urination; a fast heart rate; swelling of fingers, hands, and feet; and intermittent rapid breathing while sleeping, with brief breath holding spells. If someone is symptomatic with altitude illness (i.e., poorly acclimatized), descent to the last elevation where they felt well should resolve the symptoms. If someone is sick at high altitude, assume it is altitude sickness until proven otherwise.

Altitude illness usually affects people traveling above 6,500 to 8,000 feet (2,400 meters); it is a spectrum of disease ranging from mild to severe acute mountain sickness (AMS), high-altitude pulmonary edema (HAPE), or high-altitude cerebral edema (HACE). Mild to moderate AMS in the continental United States is most common. Remember that altitude illness may progress from an annoying headache, to debilitating sickness, to even fatal HACE. So early symptom recognition and evacuation to lower altitudes for moderate to severe disease may avoid a later rescue for a victim unable to walk or respond. There are many prescription medications for both prevention and treatment of altitude sickness.

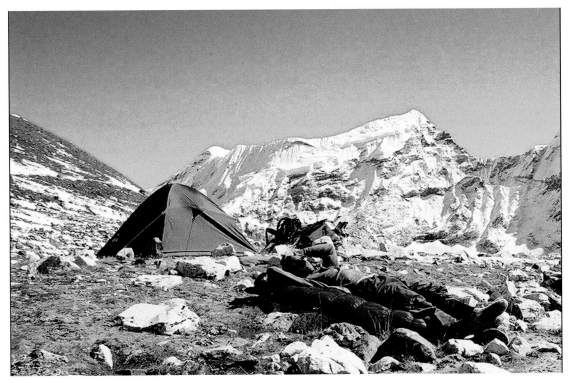

By paying attention to symptoms of altitude illness, a person can tell when they should stop ascending or descend to lower altitudes. A headache and fatigue may be early signs of acute mountain sickness. *Credit: Grant Lipman*

The most common prescription drug and considered the "gold standard" for both prevention and treatment of AMS is acetazolamide (Diamox). The drug is presumed to work by increasing the amount of urination, causing a compensatory increase in breathing and subsequent increase in the amount of delivered oxygen. The prevention dose is 125mg, twice per day; and the treatment dose for AMS is 250mg, twice per day. (Always follow the

SCOUTING GUIDE TO WILDERNESS FIRST AID

directions on the instruction label). Acetazolamide is no substitute for safe ascent profiles, as many people get AMS while taking preventive doses of the drug if they go up too high too fast. If a person has mild to moderate symptoms of AMS, they can be treated with acetazolamide and stay at the altitude they are at. No one should be treated and continue to ascend until the AMS symptoms have resolved. If symptoms are severe or there is concern that evacuation may become difficult (from deteriorating weather or other reasons), it is best to descend to the last elevation the person felt well at. Once the AMS symptoms have resolved, the individual can ascend, taking the prevention dosage of acetazolamide if they are so inclined.

Ibuprofen is a common drug (600mg taken three times a day for one day, starting the morning of ascent) that has been shown to be very effective at preventing AMS. This drug has been rigorously studied at altitudes found in North America or Western Europe, and works well at these altitudes. Likely not as efficient as acetazolamide, but the ease of over-the-counter access and low side effect profile make it an attractive option. However, it should not be used for AMS prevention at elevations above 13,000 feet (4,000 meters), like those found in the mountains of Alaska, South America, or Asia.

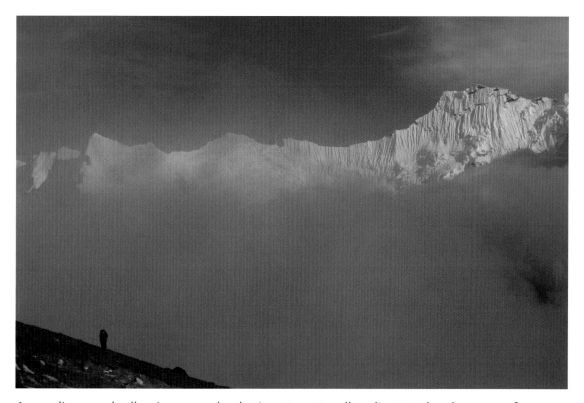

Ascending gradually gives your body time to naturally adjust to the decrease of oxygen per breath in the environment. *Credit: Grant Lipman*

Another prescription drug that is used for treatment of AMS and HACE is a steroid called dexamethasone. It is a powerful anti-inflammatory, and should never be used during ascent. Unlike acetazolamide, it does not assist with acclimatization, and may mask symptoms of altitude illness. So, if a person has taken dexamethasone (per the instruction label), it is prudent to stay at the altitude they are at for at least twenty-four hours to ensure they are asymptomatic before ascending (for moderate AMS), or to immediately descend (HACE and severe AMS).

High altitude cerebral edema presents as a severe form, or end stage, of AMS. There is progressive swelling in the brain that leads to severe headache and eventually altered level of responsiveness (LOR) that may present as confusion, amnesia, drowsiness, or unconsciousness. Another hallmark of the disease is ataxia, a gait imbalance that may present as inability to walk a straight line or loss of balance. HACE may arise as a progression of AMS symptoms, or in fulminant cases, present as a rapid neurologic deterioration without preceding symptoms of AMS. Dexamethasone and acetazolamide should be given, along with immediate descent. The person suffering for HACE should not be allowed to re-ascend, and as they are altered and unsteady, do not let them descend alone.

High altitude pulmonary edema is a disorder which presents with severe shortness of breath arising from an accumulation of excess fluid in the lung tissues and gas exchange spaces. Symptoms usually begin two to three days after ascent to high altitude, with progressive shortness of breath, cough, weakness on minimal exertion and fatigue. With greater accumulation of fluid there is severe shortness of breath, rapid heart rate, and a progressive cough that can become frothy or bloody with crackling or wheezing sounds. The person with HAPE needs to be recognized early, and descended to the last elevation they felt well at. Minimizing the amount of exertion will decrease the symptoms, so rest, backpack removal, or being carried (and oxygen if available) is ideal. Do not let this person descend alone. A decrease in as little as one thousand feet (three hundred meters) can lead to an improvement of symptoms. Once asymptomatic, the HAPE patient can (cautiously) re-ascend.

Guidelines for Safe Travel at High Altitude:

- Ascend gradually to allow time for your body to naturally compensate to the physiologic stress of a lower oxygen environment.
- When traveling above 10,000 feet (3,300 meters), do not increase sleeping altitude by more than 1,650 feet (500 meters) each night.
- For every 3,300 feet (1,000 meters) gained in sleeping elevation, take a rest day.

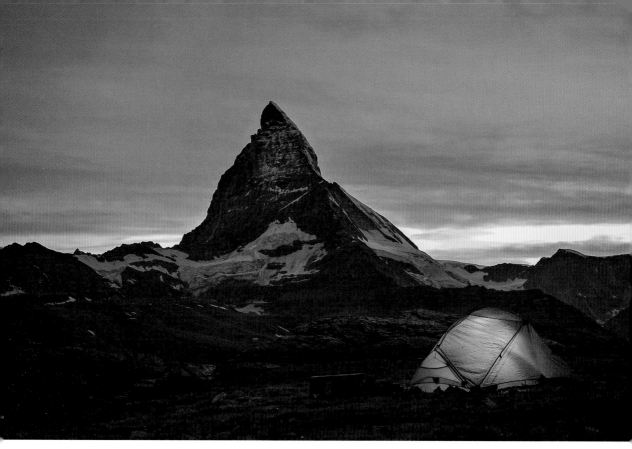

Don't increase sleeping altitude more than 1,650 feet each night when traveling at altitudes higher than 10,000 feet.

- If you feel sick at high altitude, assume it is altitude illness until proven otherwise.
- If you have mild symptoms at high altitude, do not ascend to a new sleeping altitude until you feel better.
- If you feel sick (mild symptoms) and are unable to feel normal (acclimatize) after twenty-four to thirty-six hours, descend to the last elevation where you felt well.
- If you feel sick (moderate to severe symptoms) at high altitude, descend to the last elevation where you felt well.
- Altitude illness is often more severe the morning after ascent. This should be taken into account when considering evacuation decisions in the afternoon or evening.

Symptoms

- **Mild AMS:** Headache, nausea or vomiting, fatigue, poor sleep, lack of appetite, dizziness—similar to an alcoholic hangover.

- **Moderate/Severe AMS:** More severe or pronounced symptoms of AMS that may be debilitating. The patient is too fatigued and dizzy to walk any distances; vomiting and horrible headaches will occur.
- **HAPE:** Shortness of breath and/or rapid heart rate at rest or with mild exertion.
  - ➢ Dry cough, worse when lying flat (early in disease).
  - ➢ Wet cough, weakness, difficulty catching breath (later in disease).
  - ➢ Often begins on the second day after ascent to high altitude.

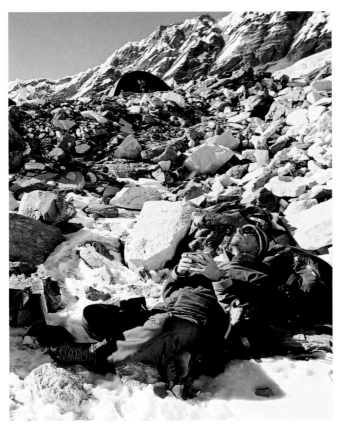

Severe shortness of breath and a cough that's worse while lying flat may be an early sign of high altitude pulmonary edema. *Credit: Grant Lipman*

- **HACE:** Altered level of responsiveness (LOR), inappropriate behavior, seizures, lethargy, or unconsciousness.
- Gait (walking) imbalance, loss of coordination.
- Severe headache.

  SCOUTING GUIDE TO WILDERNESS FIRST AID

⚠ Red Flags: Severe "ice pick" or "throbbing" headache on ascent, vomiting, any altered level of responsiveness, persistent elevated heart rate or breathing rate at rest.

Treatment

- **Mild AMS:** Maintain adequate hydration and nutrition.
  - ➤ Ibuprofen for headache (as directed by instruction label).
  - ➤ Do not ascend while feeling unwell.
  - ➤ Do not begin ascending until symptoms have completely resolved.
  - ➤ If symptoms do not improve in twenty-four to thirty-six+ hours, descend to last elevation where you felt well.
- **Moderate/Severe AMS:** Same as for mild AMS.
  - ➤ Immediate descent (at least one thousand feet or until patient feels better).
  - ➤ If possible, do not wait until morning for descent.

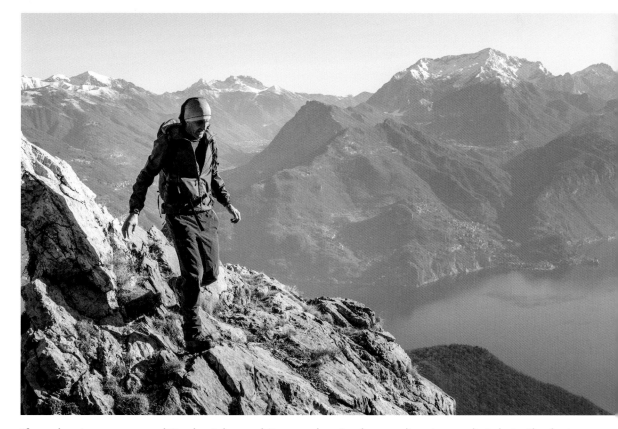

If moderate or severe altitude sickness hits you, begin descending immediately to the last elevation you felt well at.

- **HAPE/HACE:** Immediate descent (at least one thousand feet or until patient feels better).
  - ➤ If possible and safe to descend, do not wait until morning, as symptoms will likely worsen overnight, and the patient may not be able to walk out on his or her own power.

 Evacuate:
- Any person who has HACE or HAPE.
- Any person with severe AMS that is not improving.
- Never allow a sick person to descend alone.

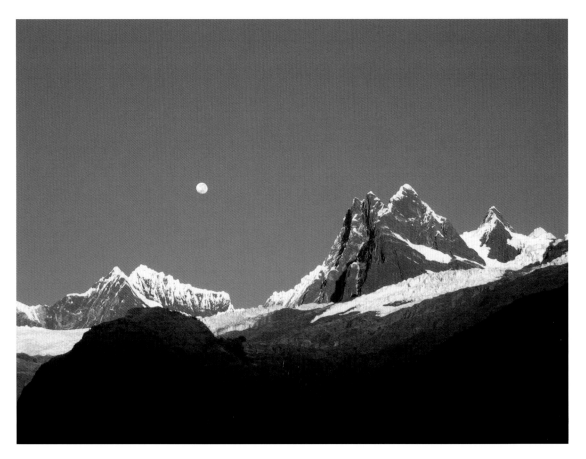

Credit: Grant Lipman

CHAPTER 5

BLISTERS

Blisters are the most commonly reported injuries in the wilderness. While preventable and easily treatable, blisters can mean the difference between an enjoyable trip and incredible discomfort.

Preparation begins with properly fitting footwear. Size the boots in the evening (when the foot is most swollen), and break them in before a trip to accustom both boots and feet to ensure comfort. Cotton socks should be avoided; a synthetic sock or a combination of thin synthetic inner sock and thicker cushioning outer sock has been shown to minimize blister occurrence. Soft and supple feet are better able to withstand the sheer stress that causes blisters than hard and cracked feet. Feet should be kept well hydrated with lotion to keep them supple, and calluses should be filed down, and toe nails kept well trimmed.

A blisters starts with a hot spot, a sensation of heat that is a warning sign that needs to be recognized and immediately treated to avoid progression to a painful blister. Treating a blister as soon as possible improves outcome and reduces potential complications. The pain of a blister arises from pressure on the incompressible blister fluid between skin layers. Small blisters that do not cause discomfort should be left intact. Otherwise, blister fluid should be drained to minimize discomfort and to keep the protective roof of the blister intact. The drainage and treatment of blisters is done in a way to minimize the possibility of infection. Blood-filled blisters represent a deeper injury, and *should not* be drained. Likewise, blisters

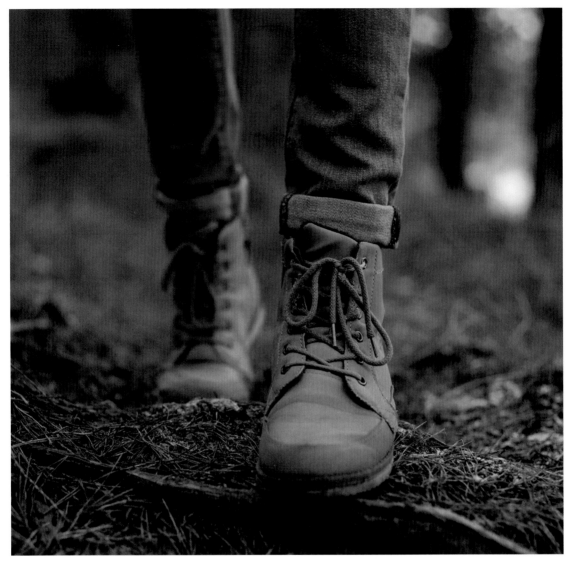

Break in boots before going on a trip to make sure that both feet will be comfortable.

underneath calluses should not be drained, as they are painful to access, may become infected, and re-accumulate fluid quickly. Keeping feet clean and dry (avoiding prolonged wetness) will lead to a lower incidence of blisters.

Symptoms: Hot Spot

- Warmth, rubbing, discomfort, pain, or raised or red area. No fluid accumulation.

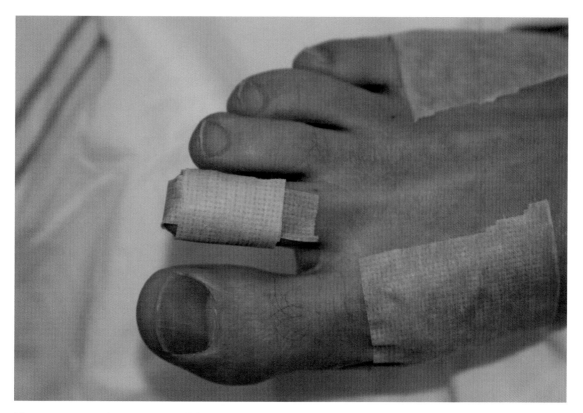

Hot spots can be prevented by pre-taping commonly irritated areas prior to starting an activity. *Credit: Grant Lipman*

Treatment

- Place a strip of paper tape over the hot spot. The length should overlap the healthy skin on either side by at least the width of the hot spot. Take care to ensure there are no "dog ears" or wrinkles, which may worsen the friction.
- **Prevention:** Apply paper tape to commonly irritated areas—pre-taping before starting your activity to prevent hot spots has been proven to be effective in preventing them.

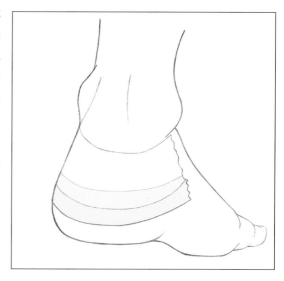

Paper tape–covered hot spot.

Symptoms: Blister

- Fluid-filled bubble of skin. Painful.

⚠ **Red Flags:** Blood-filled blister, redness/streaking around blister, blisters beneath a callus.

Treatment

- Prepare both the blister skin and safety pin with an alcohol pad (the diameter of the safety pin is larger than a sewing needle to allow continuous drainage, yet not too large as to risk de-roofing the blister).
- Puncture blister with pin at several points on the blister wall (toward the outside of the foot), rather than one large hole. This will allow natural foot pressure to continually squeeze out fluid. One large hole may destroy the integrity of the blister's roof.
- Gently push fluid out with your fingers or gauze.
- Blot expressed fluid.
- Cover with paper tape (protects the blister roof when removed), overlapping blister by double its diameter on either side.
- Can cover with benzoin (for adhesion), then shaped adhesive tape (such as Elastikon) overlapping the paper tape (twice the diameter of the blister). Trim tape with rounded corners to minimize dog-ears and rolling off.
- Re-accumulated fluid can be drained through intact bandage.

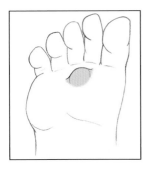
Blister.

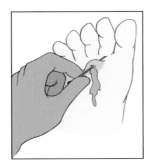
Draining a blister.

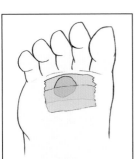
Paper tape covering a drained blister.

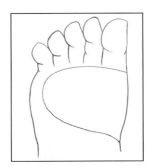
Elastikon tape covering a drained blister.

Symptoms: Open/Torn Blister

Treatment

- Using small scissors, carefully unroof the blister (painless), completely trimming off the dead skin.
- Place Spenko 2nd Skin to cover the raw area.
- Cover with paper tape.
- Can cover with benzoin (for adhesion), then shaped adhesive tape (such as Elastikon) overlapping the paper tape (twice the diameter of the blister).
- Trim tape with rounded corners to minimize dog-ears and rolling off (as discussed with regular blisters).

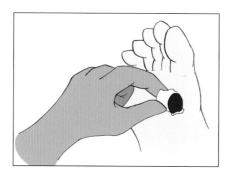

Unroofing a torn blister.

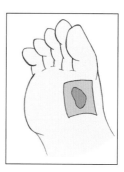

Spenko 2nd Skin–covered open blister.

Symptoms: Heel Blister

Treatment

- Treat open or closed blister as described in the steps above.
- Shape the "heel cup" by taking a length of Elastikon (or other adhesive) tape, cutting two midline incisions from either end, almost meeting in the middle, leaving a middle piece of tape intact. Looks like an *H* on its side.
- Trim all the corners.
- Apply benzoin for optimum adhesion.
- Apply the upper strip of the heel cup horizontally over the blister and intact skin above it.
- Wrap the lower two "wings" of the heel cup from under the heel up and perpendicular to the blister, with tension anchoring the wrap.
- Round off any corners or dog-ears with scissors.

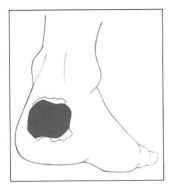

Heel blister.

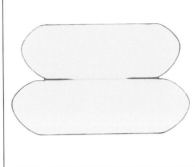

Elastikon tape cut for a heel cup.

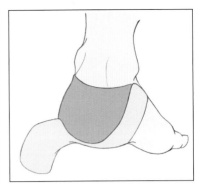

Wrapping the "wings" of a heel cup.

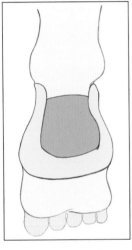

Completed heel cup.

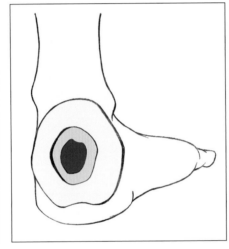

(Left) Moleskin "donut." Moleskin or Molefoam can be used on heel blisters to augment protection from a large blister. Cut a hole in the center slightly larger than the size of the blister, forming a donut shape, and place over the blister. Continue with all the steps of the above blister treatment.

Symptoms: Toe Blisters

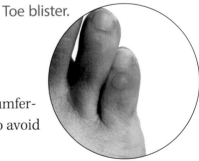

Toe blister.

Treatment

- Drain blister with prepared safety pin.
- Use one piece of paper tape to encircle the toe circumferentially (leaving tape end on top or bottom of toe to avoid irritating neighboring toes).
- Pinch closed.
- Trim sharp edges or wrinkles.
- Avoid cloth tape or Elastikon on toes, as abrasive tape will affect neighboring toes.

Evacuate: Few blister injuries require evacuation unless they are so painful that the person can't walk, or there are signs of an aggressive, spreading infection (pain with redness, streaking, pus from wound and/or fever).

Symptoms: Blister Under Toenail (Subungual Hematoma)

- Swollen, painful toe nail, with fluctuance at nail base.

Treatment

- Take an 18-gauge hypodermic needle held perpendicular to the nail area of greatest fluctuance.
- Rotate back and forth between thumb and first finger, applying downward pressure.
- Continue until blood oozes freely.
- If painful, stop.
- Put pressure on nail to squeeze out excess fluid.
- Recap needle; can reuse, as these tend to recur.
- Wrap with paper tape like a toe blister.

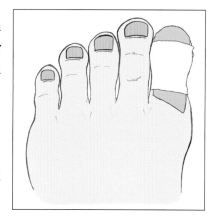

Toe blister wrapped with paper tape. Note that toe pre-taping or hot spots can be wrapped the same way.

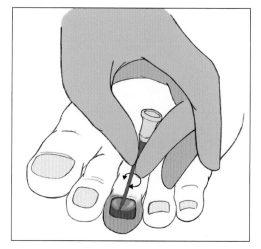

How to drain a subungual hematoma.

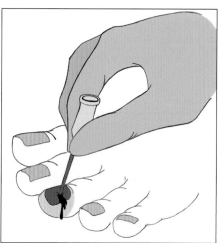

Draining a subungual hematoma.

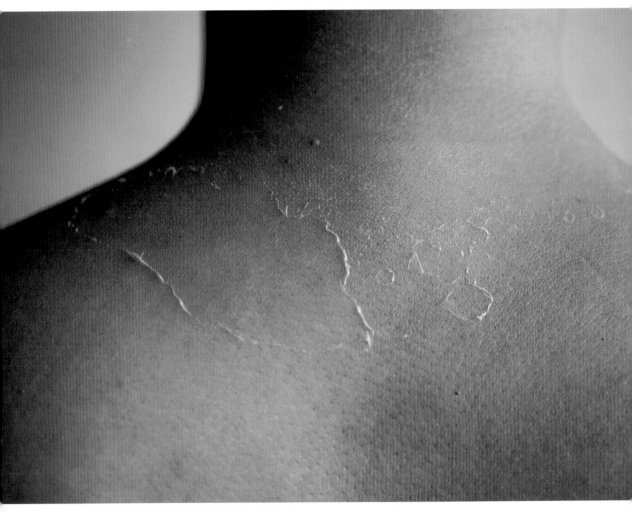

Sunburns are the most common kind of burn encountered in the wilderness.

CHAPTER 6

BURNS

The most common burn in the wilderness is sunburn. Sunburn can be avoided by wearing hats and protective clothing, and by using high SPF sunblock with frequent reapplication. Both water and snow are surfaces which refract light and can worsen sunburns. Be especially cautious at high altitude, as ultraviolet light is increased by 4 percent to 6 percent every thousand feet (three hundred meters) in elevation.

Even small burns can be painful and debilitating and larger burns may predispose the victim to dehydration. Rapid cooling of the burnt area will minimize the amount of tissue damage, but avoid ice which can cause frostbite and damage the skin more. Burns can be divided into three categories depending on the extent or severity of the burn. *First-degree burns* involve the most superficial layer of the skin. It may be painful, but there are no blisters. If there is a large area of first-degree burn the victim may feel feverish and weak. *Second-degree burns* involve the next deeper layer of skin, with blister formation and more severe pain. *Third-degree burns* involve the full thickness of the skin and may be painless as nerves have been charred. There are no blisters and the skin may be white or hard. Third-degree burns will likely be ringed by second-degree burns, which are extremely painful. First- and

Avoid sunburns with high SPF sunblock.

second-degree burns are called *partial thickness burns,* and third-degree is a *full thickness burn* that usually requires a skin graft for healing.

Like all wounds in the backcountry, burns have the potential to become infected. Large burns should be considered for early evacuation for wound care, prevention of infection, and dehydration. Blisters can be left intact if they are not at risk for spontaneous rupturing. If large and fluctuant or possibly infected (turbid and filled with milky fluid), they should be carefully drained (*see* **Blisters**). Evaluate the lungs and breathing for any difficulties breathing that may represent a burn to the airway. Measure the size of a burn with your hand (palm of hand = approximately 1 percent of total body surface area), or per body surface area involved.

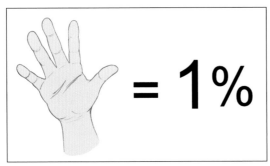

(Left) Estimation of the burn size with the palm of hand.

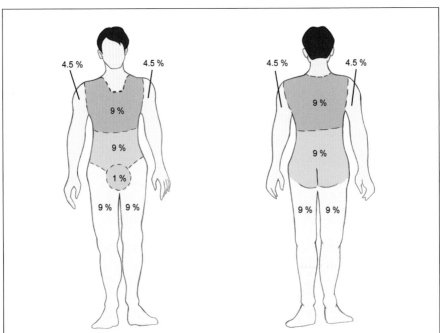

Estimation of the burn size by body surface area.

  SCOUTING GUIDE TO WILDERNESS FIRST AID

Symptoms

- **Superficial:** Reddened skin and pain (similar to a sunburn).
- **Partial Thickness:** Red skin and blistered, skin may be pale white/yellow, severe pain.
- **Full Thickness:** Flesh may be charred, no pain (nerve endings are burned).

⚠ **Red Flags:** Burns involving the face, mouth, airway, neck, hands, feet, or genitals.

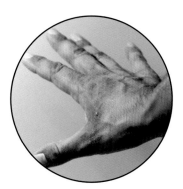

First-degree burn.

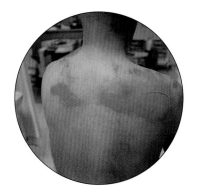

Second-degree burn.

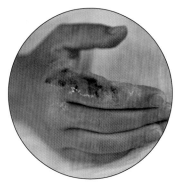

Third-degree burn.

Treatment

- Ensure the scene is safe.
- Extinguish burning clothes or material.
- Remove constricting clothes/jewelry.
- Immediately soak or copiously flush the burn with cool water (ideally for fifteen to twenty minutes).
- Wash burns with soap and drinkable water.
- Dress burn with antibiotic ointment (such as Polysporin) and nonstick gauze.
- Cover blisters with gauze dressing.
- Elevate involved extremity (to minimize swelling).
- Motrin or Tylenol for pain, per the instruction label.
- Aggressive hydration.
- Monitor for infection (change bandage every day, observe for redness/streaking/pus from wound).

 Evacuate:

- Partial thickness burns involving more than 10 percent body surface area.
- Any full thickness burn.

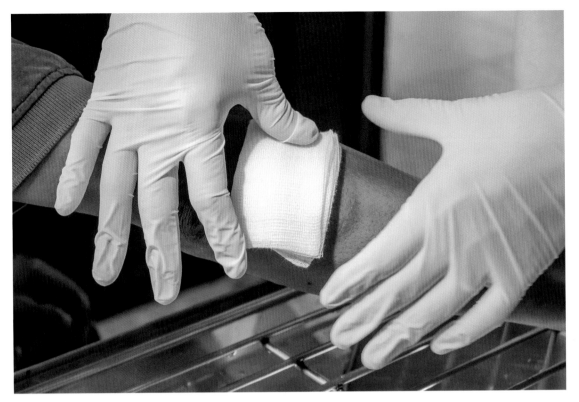

After washing the burns, dress them with antibiotic ointment and nonstick gauze.

- Any burn to the mouth, face, neck, genitals, and/or full circumference of any extremity: fingers, hands, or feet.
- Any burn that may have involved the airway (smoke inhalation), patient with cough, wheeze, singed nasal hair, or soot in nose or mouth.

CHAPTER 7

CARDIOPULMONARY RESUSCITATION (CPR)

To check for unresponsiveness and establish the need for CPR, attempt to make verbal contact in a clear and loud voice. If unsuccessful, touch the shoulder gently and repeat. If there is a need to perform CPR on someone who is not breathing, the American Heart Association recommends initiating chest compressions without checking for pulses. Open the airway using the head-tilt/ chin-lift procedure to ensure the tongue is not blocking the airway (*see* **Primary Assessment**). If there is no spontaneous breathing and the victim is unconscious, begin chest compressions.

The standards for performing CPR are well established by the American Heart Association. While CPR can be an effective life-sustaining intervention in the short term, the victim's survival rate after more than twenty minutes of CPR is very low. While CPR should be initiated when indicated, early alerting of EMS

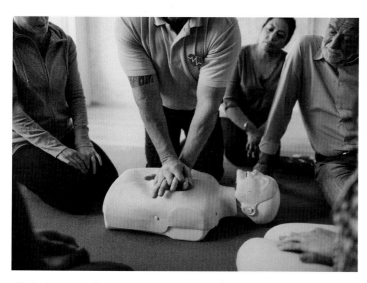

CPR classes allow you to practice proper technique with a mannequin.

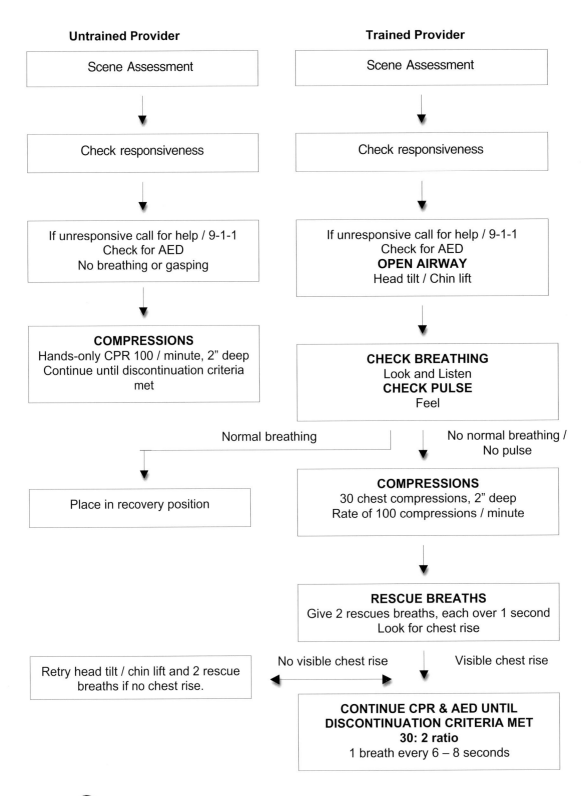

Untrained Provider

Scene Assessment

↓

Check responsiveness

↓

If unresponsive call for help / 9-1-1
Check for AED
No breathing or gasping

↓

COMPRESSIONS
Hands-only CPR 100 / minute, 2" deep
Continue until discontinuation criteria met

Normal breathing

↓

Place in recovery position

Trained Provider

Scene Assessment

↓

Check responsiveness

↓

If unresponsive call for help / 9-1-1
Check for AED
OPEN AIRWAY
Head tilt / Chin lift

↓

CHECK BREATHING
Look and Listen
CHECK PULSE
Feel

No normal breathing /
No pulse

↓

COMPRESSIONS
30 chest compressions, 2" deep
Rate of 100 compressions / minute

↓

RESCUE BREATHS
Give 2 rescues breaths, each over 1 second
Look for chest rise

No visible chest rise   Visible chest rise

Retry head tilt / chin lift and 2 rescue breaths if no chest rise.

↓

CONTINUE CPR & AED UNTIL DISCONTINUATION CRITERIA MET
30: 2 ratio
1 breath every 6 – 8 seconds

SCOUTING GUIDE TO WILDERNESS FIRST AID

for definitive care if possible is of utmost importance. These CPR protocols are not intended to be comprehensive and are no substitute for taking a CPR class, and every wilderness first responder should consider getting certified in CPR. While there are some exceptions to the rule in lightning, drowning, and hypothermia, CPR in the wilderness is rarely successful.

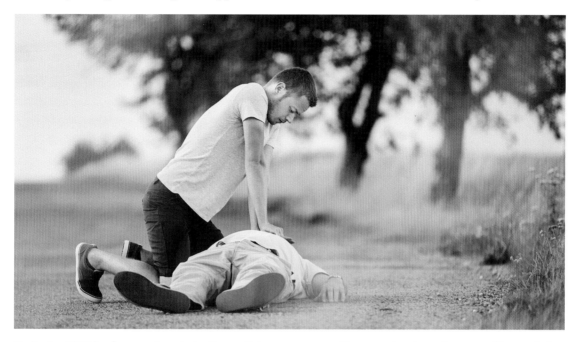

Train in CPR before going into the wilderness—you'll never know when you'll need the training.

Contraindications to CPR in the Wilderness

- Do not initiate CPR if there is:
  - ➢ Patient responsiveness.
  - ➢ Danger to rescuers, such that initiating CPR would put the rescuers at risk of harm.
  - ➢ Obvious lethal injury (i.e., decapitation).
  - ➢ A well-defined "Do Not Resuscitate (DNR)" status.

Discontinuation of CPR in the Wilderness

Once initiated, CPR should be continued until (any one of the following):

- Patient is responsive.
- The rescuers are exhausted.

- The rescuers are placed in danger.
- Patient care is turned over to EMS for definitive care.

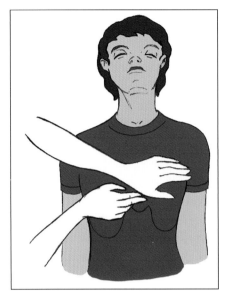

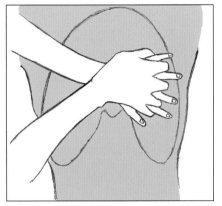

Hand position on the body for CPR.   Hand position for CPR.

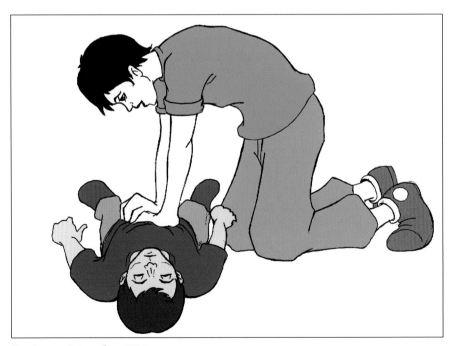

Body position for CPR.

CHAPTER 8

CHEST PAIN

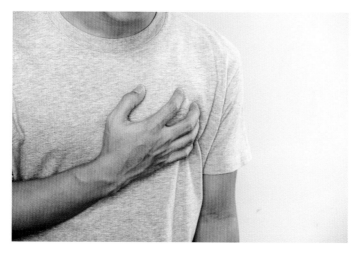

Do not ignore persistent chest pain; it could be a sign of a major issue.

Differentiating the causes of chest pain or chest pressure is challenging in the wilderness, Chest pain can be a benign infection from a viral irritant, which is often a sharp pain and reproducible when pushing on the chest wall. It may be a more serious (and potentially fatal) problem in the lungs like a blood clot (pulmonary embolism). Women on birth control are especially at risk for this, which may present gradually or suddenly, with sharp chest pain, worse on inspiration with shortness of breath—often exacerbated by lying down or exertion. Ask the patient if there is a history of heart disease or blood clots (or family history of this), or if they are currently taking medicine for high blood pressure. If so, assist them with taking the prescribed medications. Younger people may complain of persistent rapid heart rate rather than pain. While it is better to avoid exerting a patient with concerning chest symptoms, it may be timelier and more advantageous to have them ambulate to assist in the evacuation. If a patient has persistent chest pain, consider not moving the patient and bringing medical care to them.

A heart attack may present with the following symptoms: chest pain, heaviness, or shortness of breath that is exacerbated with exertion. Radiation of pain to the neck, left arm, or back, possibly with sweating and clammy skin. This is due to an inadequate supply of oxygenated blood to the heart muscle from an obstructed or narrowed blood vessel (artery) in the heart. The chest pain may be stress on the heart (ischemia) or cell death (infarction). This is difficult to differentiate in the wilderness, so assume the worst case scenario. Allowing the person to rest will minimize the stress on heart, and exerting them further will exacerbate the heart's oxygen demand and may lead to further damage to the heart muscle. Death from a heart attack is usually caused by an irregular heart beat that cannot sustain life, or a weakened muscle that cannot adequately pump blood. Early symptom recognition and prompt evacuation will hopefully minimize the chances for a bad outcome.

In some rare cases the large vessel (aorta) leading from your heart can have a tear in it. This is an aortic dissection, and is more common in people with a history of high blood pressure. The classic symptoms are a tearing intense pain, with a rapid onset and peak that radiates into the chest. While this may be challenging to differentiate from a heart attack, it requires prompt evaluation by a doctor and evacuation to definitive medical care.

Sometimes a person's heart can beat in a very rapid rate that may be in a regular or irregular rhythm. This rapid heart rate (tachycardia) may occur due to heat illness, exertion, high altitude, trauma, or pain. If the tachycardia occurs suddenly without exacerbating events, it is likely primarily a heart problem. The symptoms include a feeling of rapid heart beating ("palpitations"), skipping beats, chest tightness, lightheadedness, or weakness. There are several maneuvers to slow down the rapid heart rate without medications, These include: taking a deep breath and while pursing one's lips, bear down hard; taking a deep breath and plunging a face into cold water; or pressing gently but firmly on closed eyelids for fifteen to twenty seconds. If unable to break this cycle, it may necessitate an evacuation.

In some cases the heart beats too slow (bradycardia), and the decreased amount of oxygenated blood to the brain can cause dizziness or even a loss of consciousness. This is usually in response to a painful event, rapid change in position, or emotional stimulus. Bradycardias are rarely a primary heart malfunction, and if due to the heart muscle malfunction, hypothermia, or rare international disease in conjunction with an elevated temperature, patient should be rapidly evacuated for further care and evaluation.

Symptoms

- Chest pain, tightness, or pressure.
- Pain radiating to the left arm or jaw.
- Weakness, nausea, shortness of breath, pale skin, and/or sweating with the pain.
- Lightheaded or dizzy.

⚠ **Red Flags:** Chest pressure that is worsened by activity, reduced by resting and/or associated with sweating. Sharp, sudden onset of chest pain with difficulty breathing.

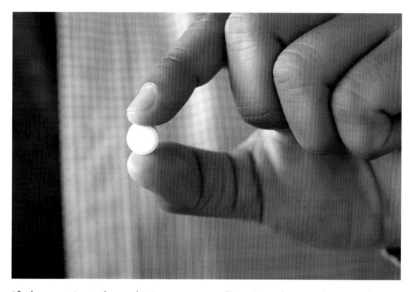

If the patient has their own medication, have them take it. Aspirin is another treatment option.

Treatment

- Reduce activity and anxiety. Place patient in a position of comfort.
- If patient has nitroglycerin, have him take his own medicine as directed.
- Give aspirin as directed by the instruction label.
- If symptoms occur at high altitude (10,000 feet plus), reduce altitude by at least 1,000 feet (300 meters).
- For younger patients with rapid heart rate, have them forcibly "hum" for thirty to sixty seconds, which can increase the firing of nerves and thus slow down the heart rate.

Evacuate:

- Any patient with chest pain worsened by exertion or persistent chest pain (twenty minutes or more).

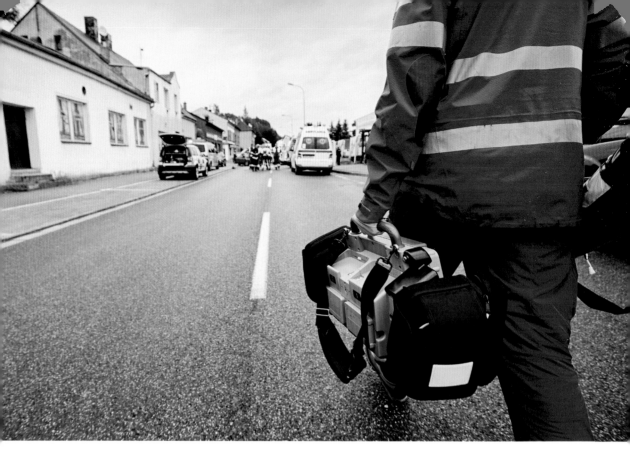

If the patient's chest pain increases with movement, try to bring EMS to them.

- Patient with persistent rapid pulse (one hundred beats per minute or more) or with associated shortness of breath and/or chest pain.
- If pain or shortness of breath is worsened by exertion, it may be of benefit to bring EMS to the patient, rather than have the patient walk out in distress.

SCOUTING GUIDE TO WILDERNESS FIRST AID

CHAPTER 9
CHEST TRAUMA

With trauma to the chest wall, force can break or bruise ribs, collapse the underlying lung, or cause bruising and bleeding in the lung. Even bruised ribs can be very painful with usually an increased amount of pain on deep inhalation. While injured ribs may make movement

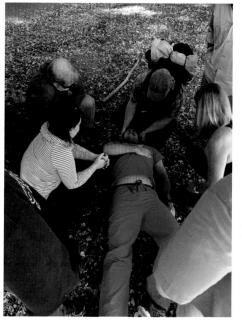

and exertion painful, the life-threatening concerns are injury to the underlying lung and blood vessels. A collapsed lung (pneumothorax) is caused by a leak of air into the potential space between the lung tissue and chest wall. As this air accumulates and expands, it exerts pressure on the lung which can then collapse with progressive pain, breathing difficulty, shortness of breath, and even collapse and death from pressure on the internal blood vessels (tension pneumothorax). Spontaneous pneumothorax can occur with a sudden complaint of difficulty breathing and/or sharp chest pain, worsened on deep breaths in the absence of

If the patient's chest is tender on touch or it is painful for them to take a deep breath, they may be experiencing chest trauma.

trauma. A bruised lung injury may have a delayed presentation of progressive shortness of breath and difficulty breathing after trauma, so careful observation is important for up to twelve hours after initial injury.

Symptoms

- Reproducible chest wall or back tenderness on touching.
- Pain on taking a deep breath.
- Sensation of being unable to take a deep breath.

⚠ **Red Flags:** Severe shortness of breath, passing out, "rice crispy" sensation over injury site, bubbles or gushing air exiting from chest wound.

Treatment

- Place the patient in a position of comfort or on the non-injured side.
- For *reproducible* rib pain, wrap painful ribs with a circumferential compression bandage (like a girdle), effectively "buddy taping" the area like you would splint a broken finger.
- Ibuprofen and acetaminophen for pain, per the instruction labels.
- Encourage patient to periodically take deep breaths (to inflate the lungs).
- If penetrating wound to chest with bubbles and/or air, affix sterile/clean gauze over wound, make an airtight seal by *taping on three sides* (leaving fourth side of bandage untaped to allow for air to exit and prevent air trapping in the lungs).

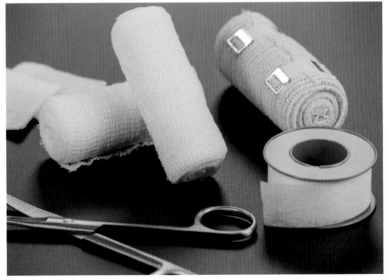

If there is a penetrating wound to the chest, use gauze and other supplies to seal the wound.

- Any symptoms of difficulty breathing or shortness of breath after chest trauma.
- Any coughing up of blood after chest injury.
- Any air bubbles/gush of air from chest wound.
- Cough producing sputum and/or fever.
- Persistent severe pain that limits ability to take comfortable breaths or walk normally, despite appropriate pain medicine and buddy taping chest wall.

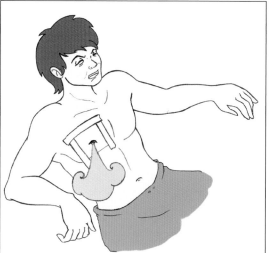

Chest trauma.

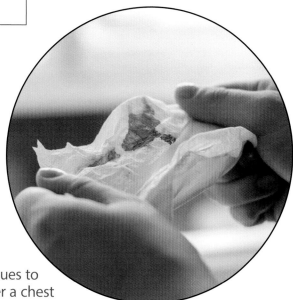

If the patient continues to cough up blood after a chest injury, you may need to evacuate.

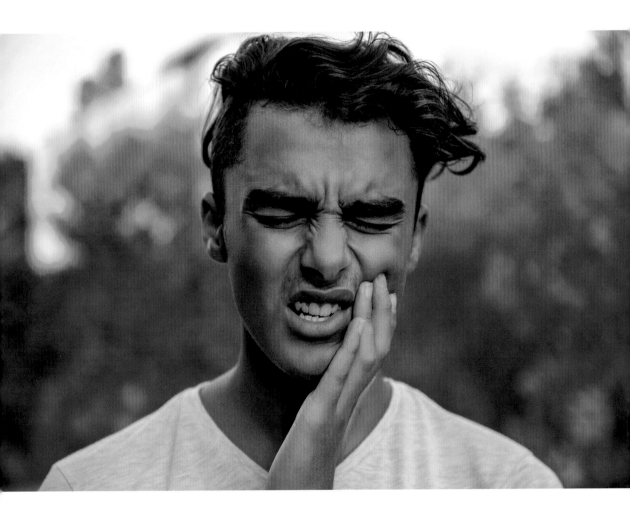

CHAPTER 10

DENTAL PAIN

Dental pain can be remarkably severe, but while potentially debilitating from discomfort, it is rarely due to a reason that will necessitate an evacuation. Tooth pain occurs in areas that have eroded due to a cavity, a traumatic injury, or a lost filling, To localize the problem tooth, tap each one individually to find the point of tenderness. If there is swelling (inflammation) to the base of the tooth or the gum and surrounding structures, the pain may be more dispersed. If there is localized gum swelling with an obvious soft and fluctuant area, this is a collection of pus called an abscess, and the drainage of this (with a cleaned needle or tip of a blade where the gum meets the tooth) will relieve some of the pressure and pain. If a tooth has been dislodged from trauma, and is partially attached, do not attempt to remove it as it could damage the root of the tooth. Rather, leave it alone and evacuate to see a dentist as soon as possible for optimal dental results. Any tooth that has been fully dislodged should not be scrubbed (which can injure the root and inhibit reattachment). Rather, gently rinse and keep moist (either between the cheek and gum if no risk of being swallowed or in a waterproof container), and be evaluated by a dentist as soon as possible for best chance at reimplantation.

It's rare that dental pain will require an evacuation, but it does help to know how to treat it.

Symptoms

- Extreme tooth sensitivity to hot or cold stimulus.
- Swelling of gum or cheek
- Visually or palpably identifiable tooth irregularity.

⚠ **Red Flags:** Severe swelling to gum or cheek with or without fever.

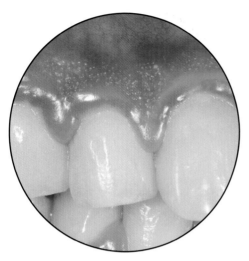

Swollen gums can be a sign of a larger problem, such as a bacterial infection.

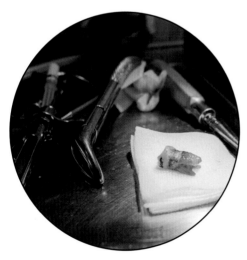

If a tooth is knocked out and cannot be replaced, do not scrub it, and wrap it in clean gauze so that a professional can replace it later.

Treatment

- If a crown or filling is lost or the tooth breaks, cover the edge or "hole" with soft candle wax or sugarless gum; bite down to get a good approximation.
- Ibuprofen and acetaminophen for pain, per the instruction labels.
- Avoid very hot or cold liquid or food. If the tooth is knocked out of the socket, irrigate the tooth with drinkable water and attempt to replace it in the socket. Do NOT scrub the roots to clean. Make a "splint" of neighboring teeth using cooled soft candle wax or dental floss tied around opposing teeth. If tooth cannot be replaced, wrap in sterile/clean gauze, and have patient carry the tooth between their cheek and gum if not at risk to be inhaled into the lungs.

🚁 **Evacuate:**

- Any patient with a tooth knocked out of the socket.
- Any broken tooth with severe pain.
- Increasing swelling to cheek or gum with or without fever.

CHAPTER 11

DIABETIC EMERGENCIES

Diabetes is a disease where the body is unable to sufficiently break down sugar. Diabetes is usually well maintained and managed in a wilderness setting. There is often an increased caloric demand during wilderness activities from an increased amount of exercise, yet insulin dose requirements often drop. The diabetic should plan with their doctor prior to embarking on a wilderness adventure. Diabetic emergencies arise because there is a mismatch between the amount of sugar (glucose) in the blood and the body's ability to utilize that sugar (too much or too little insulin). Diabetics in a wilderness setting should consider checking their blood sugar with frequency, as well as familiarizing the trip leader or colleagues with personal testing apparatus, medicines, and ensuring their trip partners are able to identify signs and treatments of low blood sugar (hypoglycemia). The diabetic should plan ahead

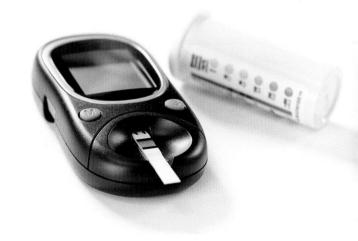

Diabetics should plan ahead and make sure to have supplies, such as a glucometer and medication, readily available.

for optimum storage and administration of supplies (glucometer; spare batteries; duplicate medications such as insulin, pills, glucose paste; syringes; and ketone strips), and establish a sick day plan. Also plan to have routine meal times.

Insulin and cold: Avoid having insulin freeze. Keep next to skin in freezing temperatures, and if frozen solid, do not thaw and use.

Insulin and heat: Avoid prolonged direct sunlight and temperatures in excess of body temperature. Store wrapped within a sock next to a cool water bottle and/or in insulated case to retain coolness. Prolonged warmth may degrade efficacy of insulin, so test sugars more frequently.

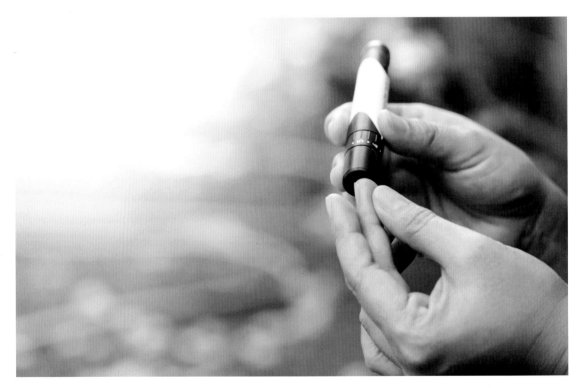

Insulin may be less efficient with prolonged heat or cold, so make sure to store insulin carefully, carry a backup supply, and to check sugar levels frequently.

Insulin should be administered by the patient only.

If unsure whether a diabetic who has an altered level of responsiveness (LOR) is suffering from too little sugar or too much, it is better to assume a low sugar state, and give sugar.

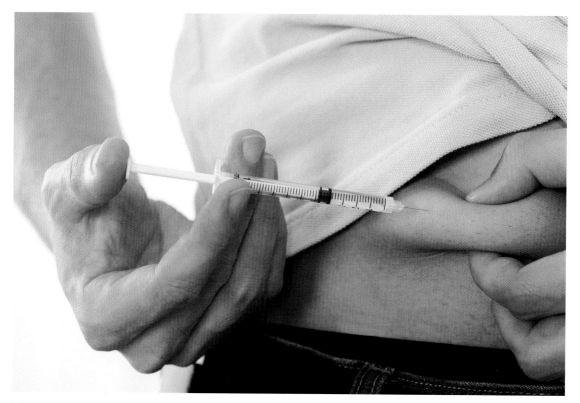

The patient should administer their own insulin.

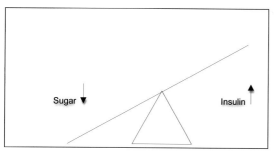

Hypoglycemia.

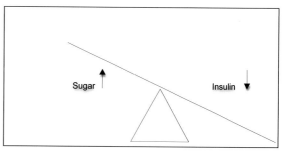

Hyperglycemia.

Symptoms

- **Low blood sugar:** Rapid onset (minutes to hours).
  - ➤ Weak, sweating, confused, slurred speech, agitated, headache, seizure. They may appear drunk.
- **High blood sugar:** Slow onset (over a day).
  - ➤ Fatigue, hunger, excessive thirst, excessive urination, abdominal pain, nausea, vomiting, weakness, or blurred vision.

➢ Possible preceding infectious symptoms.

⚠ **Red Flags:** Change in level of responsiveness, increasing thirst and/or urination.

Treatment
- Low Blood Sugar (under 60 mg/dL)
  - ➢ Check blood sugar using the patient's glucometer.
  - ➢ If conscious, give sugar/sugar water/candy, then complex carbohydrates such as a sandwich.
  - ➢ If unconscious, rub sugar/sugar containing gel on inside of cheek or under the tongue.
  - ➢ Once patient regains consciousness, give food to maintain normal blood sugar levels (80–120 mg/dL).

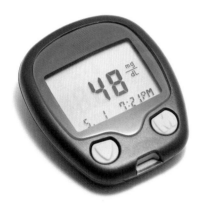

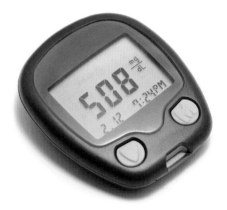

If a patient has low blood sugar, give them some sugar and carbohydrates so they can reach and maintain normal sugar levels.

If they have very high blood sugar, then they need to hydrate and evacuate.

- High Blood Sugar (over 300 mg/dL)
  - ➢ Check blood sugar using the patient's glucometer.
  - ➢ Aggressive hydration and evacuation.

 Evacuate:
- Any patient with diabetes who has lost consciousness or has prolonged changes in level of responsiveness for more than one hour.
- Persistent vomiting or diarrhea.
- Any diabetic patient who cannot (or will not) moderate his or her blood sugar levels.

SCOUTING GUIDE TO WILDERNESS FIRST AID

CHAPTER 12

DROWNING

Drowning is an event when the airways inhale (aspirate) water with subsequent breathing impairment. Drowning outcomes range from no disease, to some breathing difficulties and disease, to death. Terms to avoid are "submersion," "immersion," "near-drowning," "dry drowning," or "secondary drowning." If water is inhaled into the lungs, symptoms present quickly and progress; they do not suddenly appear days later. There is not a difference in salt-water versus fresh-water drowning, as it is the amount of water entering the lungs that produce symptoms. Always consider a traumatic injury (and possible spinal injury) in drowning victims if they have lost consciousness after diving into the water, as spinal precautions may be warranted.

In the event of a drowning resuscitation, do not attempt to push the water out through Heimlich or abdominal thrusts like you would a choking victim. Rather, approach the resuscitation like you would with anyone requiring CPR. However, in drowning the heart has usually stopped beating because of a lack of oxygen (asphyxia) in the lungs. Because this is typically a respiratory arrest that has caused a lack of a heart beat and pulse, rescue breathing should be started promptly, even while the victim is in shallow water. Resuscitations and CPR may have better outcomes in drowning than a primary cardiac (heart) event. There have been complete and successful resuscitations in cold water drownings due to hypothermia, so CPR should be continued for longer periods in such situations.

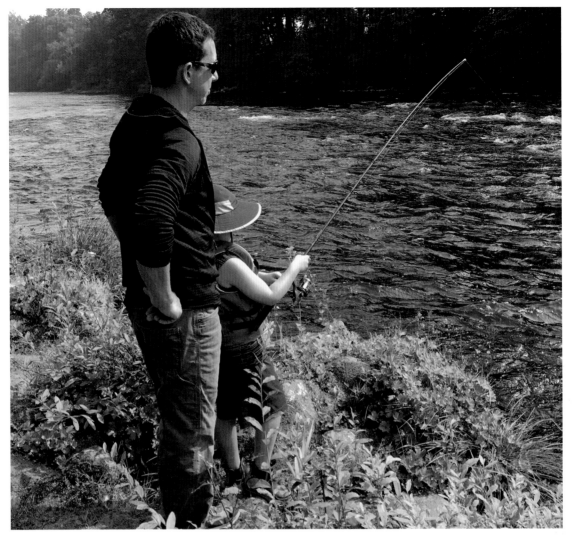

Make sure an adult is supervising any activities by the water. *Credit: Grant Lipman*

Safety and Prevention

- All water-related activities should be supervised by a responsible adult.
- It only takes seconds to inhale small amounts of water and a child can drown in seconds when an adult is not looking.
- Utilize the "buddy system"—do not swim alone.
- Be aware of weather conditions; if strong winds or thunderstorms and lightning are in the area, get out of the water and seek shelter.
- Be aware of waves and rip currents. If you are caught in a rip current and being taken

away from the beach, swim parallel to the shore until you are free from the current, then swim toward the shore.

- Everyone involved in a boating activity should wear a properly fit life jacket. A flotation toy is not an appropriate substitute.

Symptoms

- Rapid breathing rate, shortness of breath, cough, wheezing, altered level of responsiveness (LOR), unconsciousness.

⚠ **Red Flags:** Any breathing difficulties, persistent coughing (more than five minutes).

Treatment

- Ensure scene safety for the rescuer.
- Get patient onto dry land.

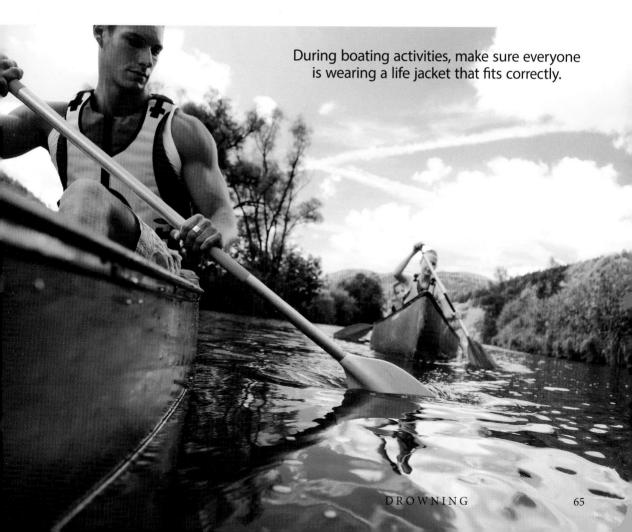

During boating activities, make sure everyone is wearing a life jacket that fits correctly.

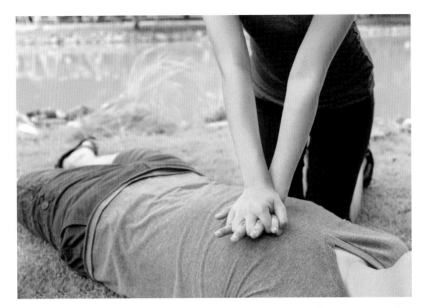

If the patient isn't breathing, initiate CPR once they are on dry land.

- Ensure spinal injury precautions if the victim was doing something that may have caused that (such as diving). (Refer to the FACS list given on page 137)
- Initiate aggressive CPR (rescue breaths and/or chest compressions) if not breathing and/or no pulse.
- Be mindful of wet clothing, and initiate hypothermia preventive care early.
- Observe for any symptoms of breathing difficulty.

Evacuate:

- Any patient who has lost consciousness.
- Any issues with breathing—persistent shortness of breath or cough, rapid breathing rate, "crackly" breathing sounds, blue discoloration around mouth—and/or altered level of responsiveness (LOR).

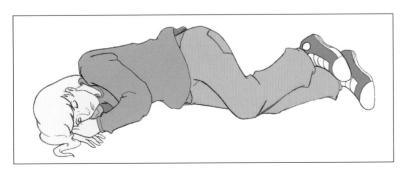

Recovery position.

SCOUTING GUIDE TO WILDERNESS FIRST AID

CHAPTER 13

EYES, EARS, NOSE, AND THROAT

Injuries and illnesses to the eyes can range from irritating to debilitating or even devastating. The most important thing with eyes is to note preceding trauma, symptom progression, and/or contact lens use. Contact lenses predispose people to more severe infections. Eye infections can be viral or bacterial and involve different depths of the eye structure. Progressive redness, a foreign body sensation, sensitivity to light, or change in visual acuity are all concerning symptoms that have limited management options in a wilderness environment, so symptoms such as these require evacuation for further care and evaluation. An infection or swelling to the eyelid (stye) should be treated with frequent (four times a day) warm compresses which can resolve it, or bring it to a head and allow it to self-drain. A foreign body lodged in the eye or underneath the eyelid is incredibly painful, but examination and eversion of the eyelid may be able to find an imbedded object, and gentle blotting may remove the offending substance. Bright and reflective surfaces such as snow, water, or sand can predispose to a sunburn to the cornea, the surface of the eye. This "snow blindness" is incredibly painful, and the pain and light sensitivity lead to a lack of vision due to inability to tolerate sunlight. Patching the eye, or cutting small slits in an eye covering, will limit the number of ultraviolet rays, decrease the pain, and make wilderness movement more negotiable. Ibuprofen for the pain is advised, and like any bad sunburn, it is self-limited and once endured is rarely repeated. Spontaneous loss of vision or visual field can be due to many reasons, from an injury to the light-receptive layers in the back of the eyeball to a problem with the blood vessels or nerves that feed the eye; regardless of the cause, loss of vision is a medical emergency that requires evacuation and emergent evaluation by an ophthalmologist.

Problems to the ears usually involve pain, trauma, change in hearing, or drainage. Ear pain (even with a fever) is usually an infection caused by a virus, which may resolve on its own without the need for antibiotics. Even a draining ear will usually resolve on its own. This is usually the same for facial/sinus pain and pressure, which is typically caused by viruses and managed by over-the-counter pain medicine.

Nose bleeds usually originate for injured blood vessels along the middle partition (septum) of the nose. Direct pressure is the best way to stop the bleed, but first the blood clot needs to be evacuated so it will not stent open the nostrils and inhibit the pressure point. After copiously blowing the nose, the victim will need to pinch the nostrils for ten to fifteen minutes. This is a long time to apply direct pressure, and it is more feasible to fashion a clothespin type apparatus by longitudinally cutting a green twig that can then be clamped over the nostrils. Nose bleeds are common in the mountains and can be due to irritation to the nasal lining by dry air. Preventive application of an antibiotic ointment or petroleum-based ointment to the nasal septum can lubricate the fragile mucosal lining and help minimize the fragile blood vessels.

Sore throats are most commonly caused by viruses. While uncomfortable, the pain, hoarse voice, swollen neck lymph nodes, and often fever is self-limited and treated with over-the-counter anti-inflammatories and salt-water gargles. In rare cases, the sore throat may represent a serious bacterial infection that may track to the deep tissues of the mouth and neck. This presents as severe pain, often with a high fever, difficulty opening the mouth, tenderness to the floor of the mouth or front of the neck, or a muffled "hot potato" voice. This needs to be evacuated.

Symptoms: Eyes
- Foreign body sensation, pain, irritation, tearing, redness, sensitivity to light.
- Severe pain/light sensitivity twelve hours after extended exposure to bright/reflected sunlight (possible snow blindness).
- Specks or "floaters" in vision.

⚠ **Red Flags:** Colored drainage from eyes, pain and redness in only one eye, loss of vision, or new "floaters."

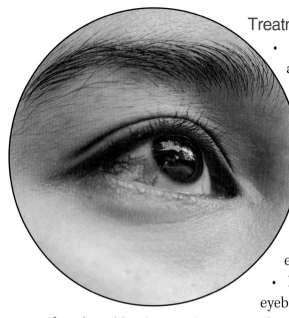

Treatment

- If foreign body sensation, irrigate with drinkable water.
  - If foreign body visualized, dab at it with moist clean cloth or cotton swab. Avoid scraping or rubbing the foreign body, as that may increase damage to the eye.
  - If painless blood to white portion of eye, do nothing. This is not dangerous.
  - If impaled object in eye, stabilize object with gauze padding and tape, and patch both eyes.
- If possible "snow blindness" (sunburn to the eyeball), patch eyes or keep covered. (If no sunglasses, consider using cloth or duct tape or a survival blanket with small slits or pinprick holes to see through). Ibuprofen and acetaminophen (as directed by the instruction label) for pain.

If you have blood or redness in one eye and it isn't painful, this is likely nothing to worry about. However, if you feel pain, it is a red flag.

Symptoms: Ears

- Ear pain, tenderness to manipulation of external ear, foreign body sensation, drainage from the ear.

Treatment

- Ear should be flushed with warm water via an irrigation syringe.
- Ibuprofen and acetaminophen for pain, per the instruction labels.

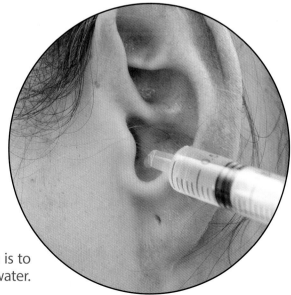

One way to treat ear pain is to flush it with warm water.

Symptoms: Nose

- Bleeding from one or both nostrils.

Treatment

- Sit patient upright, then blow both
  nostrils hard to evacuate the clot.
  Pinch and hold the nose at the
  nostril crease. Hold constant pressure for fifteen minutes. If unable
  to control bleeding, consider packing the nose with gauze (soak gauze
  in regular (non-herbal) tea to assist
  with constriction of the blood vessels).
- If mild nose bleed that stops on its own,
  consider applying antibiotic ointment inside
  nostril to lubricate; otherwise dry skin may
  be irritated and at risk for rebleeding.

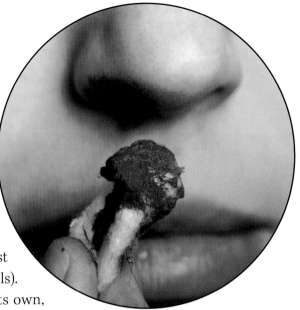

If unable to stop a nose
bleed, one option is to pack
the nostril with gauze.

Symptoms: Throat

- Pain to throat, hoarse voice, swollen neck lymph nodes.

Treatment

- Take Motrin, gargle with warm water or salt water.

⚠ **Red Flags:** Pain when opening the mouth, pain to the floor of the mouth or front of the
neck, persistent high fevers.

🚁 **Evacuate:**

- Persistent eye pain, purulent discharge, severe redness to both eyes, or any changes
  in visual acuity to one or both eyes.
- Eye redness/foreign body sensation in a contact lens wearer (which may signify a
  dangerous infection).
- Impaled object in the eye. Patient will have eyes patched and be unable to see or
  ambulate. Will need to bring EMS to the patient.
- Persistent nosebleed or nosebleed that requires packing.
- Throat pain with difficulty swallowing, severe pain making it difficult to swallow
  liquids or food, or a muffled voice.

CHAPTER 14

FEMALE GENITAL PROBLEMS

If a woman has a genital problem in the wilderness, diagnosis and treatment is often based solely on a patient's history. It is of primary importance to determine if any female with lower abdominal pain and/or vaginal bleeding is pregnant, as this will necessitate an emergent evacuation to ensure the symptoms are not due to an ectopic pregnancy (an embryo that develops outside the uterus) which is a medical emergency. Severe pelvic pain may be due to twisted ovaries that impinge on the blood supply (torsion), a surgical emergency. Excessive or irregular bleeding may be due to changes in exercise and exertion, and after a negative pregnancy test to ensure no ectopic pregnancy, menstrual flow is best contained with a tampon (if the patient is experienced and comfortable with this technique). Vaginal discharge or itching may be due to humidity and changes in the vaginal flora rather than an infection, and as gynecologic evaluation is unfeasible, any copious discharge or severe pain should be evaluated by definitive medical care.

Symptoms: Vaginal Bleeding

- Vaginal bleeding, painful menstrual cramps, bilateral or middle lower abdominal pain, pain two weeks after last menstrual period.

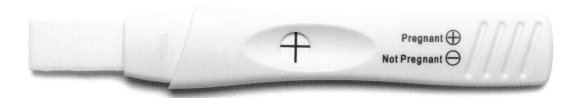

When vaginal bleeding occurs, it is important to determine if the patient is pregnant. This will help determine if evacuation is necessary.

Treatment
- Pregnancy test.
- Motrin or Tylenol (as directed by instruction label) for pain.
- Hot water bottle to abdomen.

Symptoms: Urinary Problems
- Burning on urination, increased frequency of urination, blood in urine.

⚠ **Red Flags:** Pain and tenderness to flank area and/or fever.

Treatment
- Aggressive hydration.

Symptoms: Vaginal Burning, Itching, Discharge

Treatment
- Wash vaginal area well, air dry well.
- Consider wearing cotton underwear, especially at night.

Symptoms: Pelvic Pain

Treatment
- Treat with Motrin every six to eight hours, per the instruction label.

🚁 **Evacuate:**
- Any pregnant patient with lower abdominal pain.
- Severe unrelenting pelvic pain.
- Any pregnant patient with vaginal bleeding.

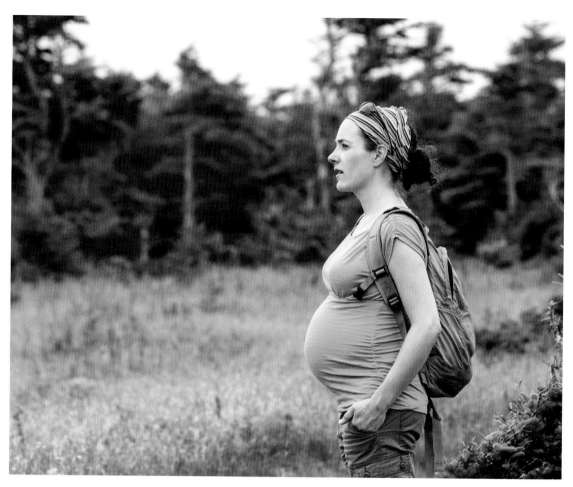

If a pregnant patient has lower abdominal pain or vaginal bleeding, it is best to evacuate.

- Symptoms of urinary problems that do not respond to supportive therapy and/or persistent fever, as the patient likely has an infection that will require antibiotics.
- Patient with pain or tenderness to flank area.

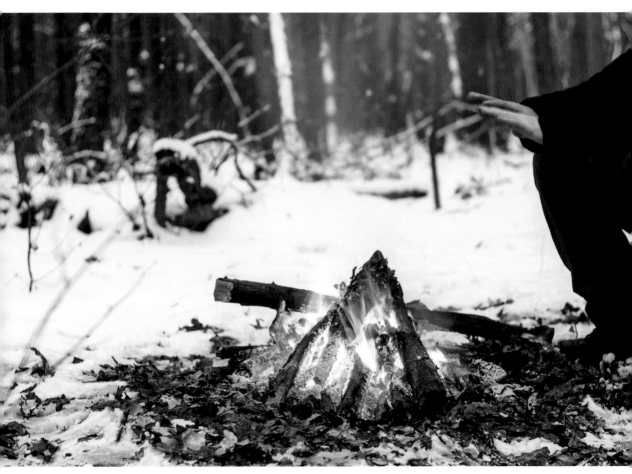

Take steps to keep the extremities warm during freezing weather to avoid frostbite.

CHAPTER 15

FROSTBITE

Cold exposure can cause both freezing and non-freezing injuries, depending on the depth of the skin layers involved. Frostnip is ice crystal formation on the superficial layers of skin, not actual skin freezing, and it leads to numb, pale or white soft skin which can be easily treated in the field. Frostbite is the actual freezing of cells that can lead to permanent tissue injury and debilitating outcomes and amputation. Extremities such as ear lobes, nose, fingers, and toes are most prone to cold injury. Factors contributing to cold injury include: hypothermia, prior frostbite, dehydration, constricting clothing/boots, wind, severity of cold environment, and concurrent alcohol or tobacco use (by adults). Cold and wet environments, cold and windy conditions, and extremely low temperatures cause the highest risks for frostbite. Care should be taken to ensure risk awareness in cold weather travelers and that numb extremities are rapidly and repeatedly evaluated for cold injury.

Frostbite typically presents with numbness due to freezing of the nerves along with the other tissue, and the skin's change to a white, waxy appearance, which may become firm or hard depending on the depth of the tissue involved. Rapid rewarming is the mainstay of therapy to decrease tissue loss, unless there is risk of refreezing, as refreezing of the thawed frostbite will cause the injured cells to be further injured, decrease the viability of affected tissue, and worsen outcomes. It is better to hike out on frostbitten toes then to thaw them in the field, and then risk refreezing the injury.

If the decision is made to rewarm frostbite in the field, protect and treat generalized cold injury (*see* **Hypothermia** section), remove constrictive clothing or jewelry, and prepare for a painful situation as the skin is thawed and sensation returns. The injured areas once rewarmed may remain numb, and should be protected against further injury with soft and fluffy bandages if available. Increased pain and bloody blisters or dark dusky skin often occur six or more hours after the initial injury, and reevaluation of the initial frostbite injury may reveal progression and severity of disease.

Frostbite severity is often staged similar to thermal burns and has been also "graded" on appearance of the frostbite lesion post-thawing, however the extent of tissue damage is usually not apparent for several days. As such, one should be conservative in estimating the seriousness of the frostbite injury and assume the worst rather than risk eventual amputation due to initial underestimation.

Grade I: Superficial/partial thickness with resolved lesion or clear blisters, tissue loss is minimal or none, and amputation is rare.

Grade II: Lesions to the distal tips of the fingers or toes.

Grade III: Lesions to fingers or toes up to the knuckle.

Grade IV: Lesions to the mid-foot or hand.

Symptoms

- Pale, white, waxy, hard skin; numbness (may feel like a "chunk of wood").
- Blanching of extremities (pinking of nail bed after pressure takes three seconds or more).
- Blisters (clear).
- Mottled, dusky, "bluish" skin.
- After re-warming, skin is swollen, red, painful.
- May develop clear blisters
- May develop blood-filled blisters (represents a deep tissue injury).

⚠ **Red Flags:** Dusky mottled skin, blood-filled blisters.

Treatment

- Primary treatment is the rapid rewarming of frozen extremity *only* if there is no risk of refreezing.
- Thaw with non-scalding water (104°F–106°F). Water should be hot-tub temperature.
- Keep affected extremity submerged for twenty to thirty minutes, or until skin becomes soft and returns to normal color (likely need to reheat water).
- Motrin (as directed by instruction label) for pain.
- Dress with clean gauze between fingers or toes and around extremity.

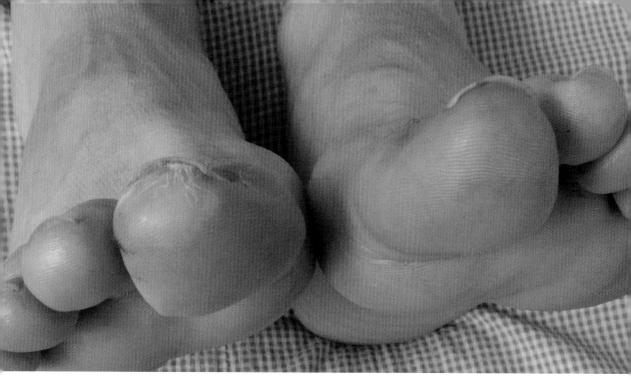

Clear blisters after rewarming are a sign of mild frostbite (Grade I).

- Do not rewarm with radiant heat (fire).
- Do not massage or rub with snow.
- Blisters: drain clear blisters if fluctuant and at risk for spontaneous rupture (*see* **Blisters**). Do not drain blood-filled blisters.

Evacuate:
- Any patient with suspected Grade II to Grade IV frostbite.
- Any patient with blood-filled blisters.
- Any patient with dusky, blotchy skin.
- Any patient unable to use the injured extremity due to either pain or immobility.
- When you are unable to protect area from further cold or refreezing.
- Any patient whose pain cannot be managed in the field.
- When there are any signs of infection to affected area.

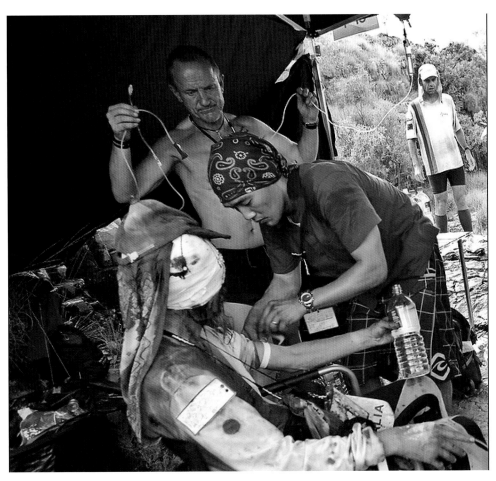

It's important to be vigilant with head injuries,
especially during the first twenty-four hours.

CHAPTER 16

HEAD INJURY

Anyone who has suffered an injury to the head is potentially at risk for progressive bleeding and swelling in or around the brain. Despite evidence of trauma with scalp bleeding or a large bump or swelling, serious sequalae to most minor head injury is rare. People who have a bleed around their brain deep inside their skull from a head injury may initially appear well and oriented, only to later decompensate with an altered level of responsiveness as the pressure inside the skull increases from the bleeding. The first few hours after a head injury are the most important to observe the patient for worsening symptoms—which may represent a more severe head injury than initially suspected that requires evacuation to medical care and possibly even neurosurgery. Delay in presenting symptoms of a severe head injury are more common in the elderly and children. Be aware of any medications such as anti-platelet drugs or blood thinning drugs (anti-coagulants) that put an individual at higher risk for bleeding and delayed presentations of severe head injury. There is no science that clearly dictates how often someone's neurologic status should be checked to ensure they are not progressing from minor to severe head injury, and if the victim falls asleep, how often they should be woken up to check their status. Immediately following a head injury, someone should not go to sleep as lethargy or somnolence is a concerning sign. But once asleep, it is reasonable to wake them every two to four hours to ensure responsiveness.

Symptoms of a concussion may be present with or without initial loss of consciousness. Always consider the mechanism of injury (MOI) for possible concurrent spinal injury and necessary spinal immobilization precautions. Scalp lacerations tend to bleed, a lot. Apply a wound dressing of gauze folded into a small square over the site of bleeding, as the smaller the surface area of bandage the greater the amount of exerted pressure. Apply compression with a circumferential bandage or compression wrap (*see the* **Wound Care** section for closure of scalp lacerations). Prevention of head injuries should focus on wearing a helmet in high risk situations, like biking, rock climbing, white water sports, or areas with potential for rockfall.

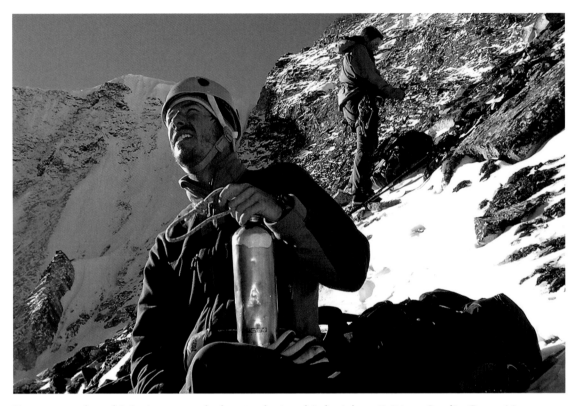

To prevent head injuries, wear helmets during high risk activities. *Credit: Grant Lipman*

Symptoms: Minor Head Injury

- Headache, transient nausea and/or vomiting, "seeing stars," dizziness, mild decrease in level or responsiveness (LOR), or appears "dazed." These symptoms should resolve quickly.

⚠ **Red Flags:** Loss of consciousness, rapid decompensation after initial injury (patient may appear drunk or have a progressive change in normal behavior).

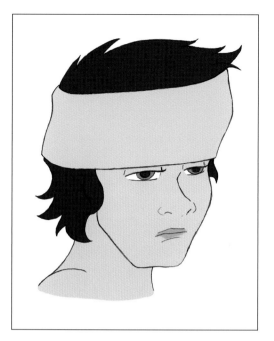

Head injury wrap.

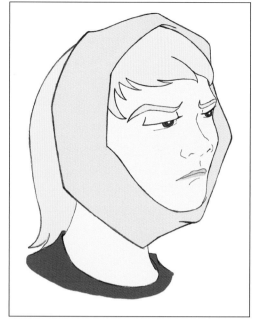

Head injury wrap.

Treatment

- Ensure that symptoms resolve quickly.
- Monitor for twelve hours to ensure no worsening of symptoms.
- Motrin or Tylenol for headache, per the directions on the instruction label.

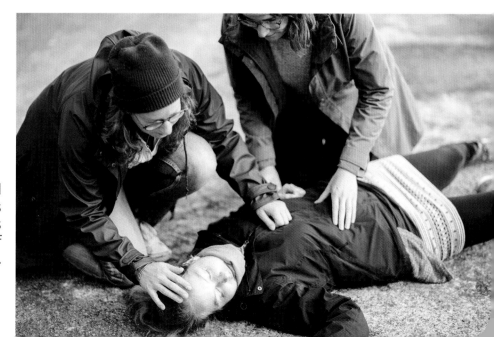

Head injury red flags include loss of consciousness or a lack of responsiveness.

Symptoms: Severe Head Injury

- Persistent symptoms of mild head injury that worsen in severity, blurred vision, lethargy, increasing disorientation, irritability, combativeness or otherwise altered level of responsiveness (LOR), persistent sleepiness, lack of coordination, seizures, persistent nausea or vomiting. There may be leaking clear fluid from the nose or ears.

⚠ **Red Flags:** Black eyes or bruising behind ears, worsening symptoms of minor head injury.

🚁 **Evacuate:**

- Any patient with progressive symptoms.
- Any patient with persistent altered LOR after head injury.
- Any patient with symptoms of severe head injury.
- Any patient whose symptoms of minor head injury do not show improvement or persistent or worsening headache after twelve hours.

CHAPTER 17

HEAT ILLNESS

Heat illness might be due to passive exposure to high ambient temperatures, overexertion in the heat, under- or over-hydration, or medications that exacerbate the body's response to a hot environment. The hotter the temperature, the more at-risk the patient is to overhydrate, which can be as dangerous (or more so) than dehydration in the heat. Over-hydration with plain water during exertion without eating salty food or consuming electrolytes may lead to a dangerous dilution of the body's salt balance (hyponatremia). Always rehydrate with electrolyte-containing fluids and/or salty foods. Individual risk factors for heat illness include: someone who is not used to hot conditions (unacclimatized), or on certain medications (some cardiac medicines, high blood pressure medicines, anti-anxiety/depressants, over-the-counter cold medicines, alcohol, stimulants). Dehydration will limit the body's ability to respond adequately to heat stress, so always begin exercising in the heat well hydrated.

A person is more susceptible to heat illness in humid conditions, as increased amount of atmospheric water vapor will minimize the vapor pressure gradient between the skin and surrounding air, inhibiting evaporation of sweat and subsequent heat loss. For example, 100°F (37.8°C) in 20 percent humidity will feel like 132°F (55.6°C) in 60 percent humidity. Heat is generated both externally through environmental exposure, and internally through exercise which can increases metabolism by twenty-five times, of which 75 percent to 80 percent is converted to heat. Heat is exchanged through four main mechanisms:

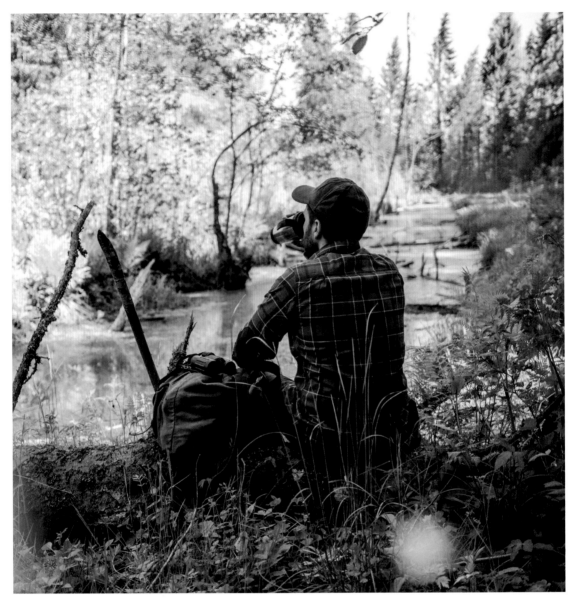

Staying hydrated may help to prevent heat illness.

Convection: Heat transferred through a gas or liquid, like air or water. When the surrounding air is warmer than approximately 91°F (33°C), heat will be gained by the body. Wind chill can cool a body.

Conduction: Heat exchange by two surfaces in direct contact. Immersion in cold water will lose heat; sitting on hot ground (or immersion in hot water) will cause heat to be gained.

Evaporation: As a liquid is phase-changed into a gas, heat is lost. For every 1.7 mL of sweat is evaporated from the skin, 1kCal of heat is lost.

Radiation: Heat transfer through electromagnetic waves. Standing in the sun is a simple example of heat gain through radiation, while the body radiates heat to cool.

Heat illness like swelling to the extremities, muscle cramps ("heat cramps"), or fainting ("heat syncope") are all self-limited. Fainting in the heat is usually due to the heat induced dilation of blood vessels and subsequent pooling of blood in the extremities. The diminished return of oxygenated blood to the brain can cause the dizziness or passing out, which has a spontaneous return to normal level of responsiveness (LOR). Anyone who loses consciousness in the heat has declared themselves poorly acclimatized to the hot conditions, and it is reasonable to observe them for a while, to ensure that they are able to eat, drink, and exert themselves comfortably.

For more severe heat illness, cold water immersion is the fastest and usually only effective way to rapidly cool someone with serious heat illness; immerse up to the level of the armpits and be cautious to keep shoulders and head dry and secure, in case of loss of consciousness. If unable to immerse the patient in a body of water, douse all clothes and head in water to optimize heat transference. Stop the cooling once normal LOR has returned. Be concerned for anyone who is hot with altered consciousness, as this is a heat stroke victim until proven otherwise, which is a life-threatening emergency and they will need to be cooled as rapidly as possible. Altered level of consciousness without elevated body temperature may be hyponatremia, so a careful and accurate patient history of recent fluid consumption and symptoms may be more helpful than a thermometer.

Symptoms: Low Salt Level (Hyponatremia)

- Weakness, nausea, dizziness, headache, fatigue, muscle cramps. May have history of decreased urine output as the body may inappropriately retain water. Symptoms may appear similar to that of heat exhaustion.
- Altered LOR (without elevated temperature), seizures, unconsciousness.

⚠ **Red Flags:** Vomiting and unable to tolerate fluids, altered LOR, seizures.

Treatment

- With mild symptoms, stop the patient from further fluid intake and the body will urinate out the excessive fluid balance. Patient should feel better.
- If tolerable, can rehydrate with a concentrated electrolyte solution or salty foods. Can

dissolve several bouillon cubes in a cup of water for a highly concentrated salty slurry.
- If any altered LOR or unable to tolerate salty fluids/foods by mouth, evacuate.

Symptoms: Heat Cramps
- Cramps of muscles, which may involve small or large muscle groups.

Treatment
- Stop exertion and rest in shade.
- Gentle stretching and massage to the painful muscles.
- Hydrate with a solution containing electrolytes.

Symptoms: Fainting
- Dizziness, nausea, loss of consciousness.

⚠ **Red Flags:** Persistent altered level or responsiveness (LOR), inability to eat, drink, or ambulate due to dizziness, concurrent symptoms of chest pain, or shortness of breath.

Treatment
- Stop exertion and rest in shade.
- Rehydrate with electrolyte-containing fluids.
- Evaporative and conductive cooling: wet the victim's clothes/head and make a fan/ draft to dissipate heat.

Symptoms: Heat Exhaustion
- Flushed, rapid pulse, sweating, dizzy, nausea, vomiting, muscle cramps, headache, chills, history of decreased fluid intake and/or urine output. May appear with symptoms similar to hyponatremia.
- Crampy abdominal pain.

⚠ **Red Flags:** Dark yellow or bloody urine, decreased urine output, too fatigued to continue, unable to tolerate fluids by mouth.

Treatment
- Stop exertion and rest in shade.
- Aggressively rehydrate with electrolyte-containing fluids.
- Gentle stretching for cramps.

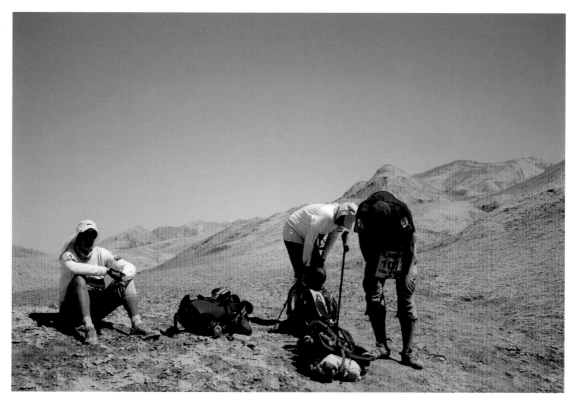

Heat exhaustion can lead to inability to continue exertions and complete immobility.

- Evaporative cooling: wet the victim's clothes/head and make a fan/draft to dissipate heat through evaporation.
- Cool with dousing of clothes, head, face, and hands with water.
- If more severe symptoms, can consider immersive cooling.

Symptoms: Heat Stroke

- Symptoms of heat exhaustion but with altered LOR and elevated temperature.
- Seizure, confusion, unconsciousness.
- Patient may be sweating or have dry skin, may be flushed or pale.

Treatment

- Similar treatment for heat exhaustion, with aggressive cooling: remove constricting and insulative clothing, cold water immersion is first choice (if available), otherwise soak the person all over with available water. Can fan to increase evaporation.

- Cautious hydration of the patient with altered LOR, as they are at risk of seizures and subsequent vomiting and aspiration.
- Cool immediately. Do not delay cooling for evacuating.

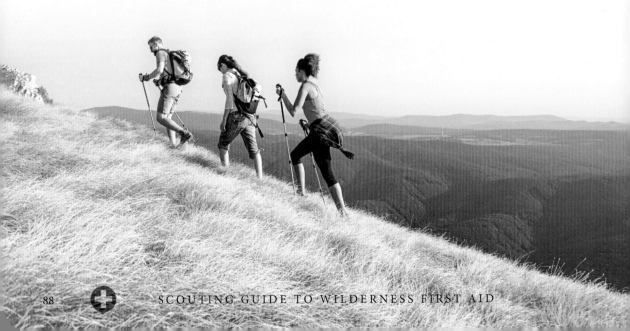 **Evacuate:**

- Heat stroke (or any altered LOR); these should have EMS brought to them to minimize exertion and further heat generation.
- Persistent symptoms of heat exhaustion that do not improve.
- Red/brown urine.

CHAPTER 18

HYPOTHERMIA

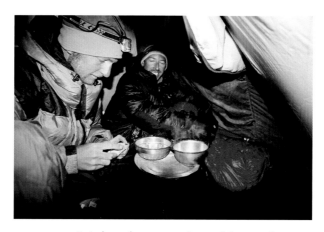

Dress appropriately when out in cold weather to avoid hypothermia and other issues. *Credit: Grant Lipman*

Hypothermia occurs when the body's ability to produce heat through metabolic activity combined with heat retention is overwhelmed by the cold effect. Heat can be lost by the same four mechanisms found in heat illness. Windy and wet conditions lead to more rapid and severe heat loss, with moisture increasing heat loss twenty-four times faster than dry. Hypothermia treatment has three main focuses: (1) to recognize the severity of presenting hypothermia; (2) increase heat production; and (3) minimize further heat loss. Synthetic clothes with multiple layers will be better able to wick sweat and remain warm when wet than organic fibers—hence the saying "cotton kills."

The Swiss have defined the severity of hypothermia (abbreviated HT) based on the presenting signs and symptoms as HT I (mild, clear consciousness with shivering); HT II (moderate, impaired consciousness that may progress to loss of shivering); HT III (severe, unconscious); HT IV (profound, apparent death); and HT V (death). Cold slows down the body's metabolic processes, with a decrease in brain metabolic rate of 6 percent to 7 percent per 2°F. So someone who is cold with normal mental function may not be hypothermic. Shivering and confusion can further be differentiated from confusion and a lack of shivering in severity of hypothermia. Awareness and recognition of these clinical stages is more important than the patient's temperature, as it may be difficult to obtain an accurate temperature measurement in the wilderness. **HT I:** Mild hypothermia can effectively be managed in the field, but any symptoms of **HT II** or worse (cold and impaired level of responsiveness) must be recognized early, as the wilderness setting offers limited interventions other than providing shelter from the wind and cold, removing wet clothing, and increasing metabolic heat production through exercise and "stoking the fire" through ingesting calories. Recognize that HT II and worse will likely require evacuation and rewarming via hospital care.

Avoid small heat packs for rewarming or body to body contact for hypothermic victims (although useful to warm cold fingers and toes). The localized heating may reduce shivering which will minimize internal heat generation, but they do not appreciably increase the rewarming rate over shivering alone. Calories are more important than a heated drink, as the heat generated from ingested calories will stoke the metabolic furnace and will be more advantageous than a warmed liquid. Consider not walking or exercising the victim for thirty minutes after starting the rewarming process, as this will avoid recirculating the cold blood to the body's core and preventing a precipitous drop in temperature. Be careful and handle HTIII/IV patients gently, as the cold heart is irritable and prone to fatal heart rhythms. Very cold people (especially after cold water drowning) have survived after prolonged arrest, so hypothermia is an exception to the regular instructed time limitations of wilderness CPR. There is a saying, "You are not dead until you are warm and dead," so CPR should be attempted on hypothermic dead-appearing patients, except in situations where there is a non-compressible frozen chest, obvious signs of death (i.e., decapitation) or an avalanche burial longer than thirty-five minutes and airway obstructed with snow.

Symptoms: HT I – Mild Hypothermia, 95°F–90°F (35°C–32°C)

- Shivering (persistent).
- Loss of fine motor coordination (stumbling).
- Withdrawn, irritability, and poor judgment (mumbling).

Treatment

- Change the environment and find shelter.

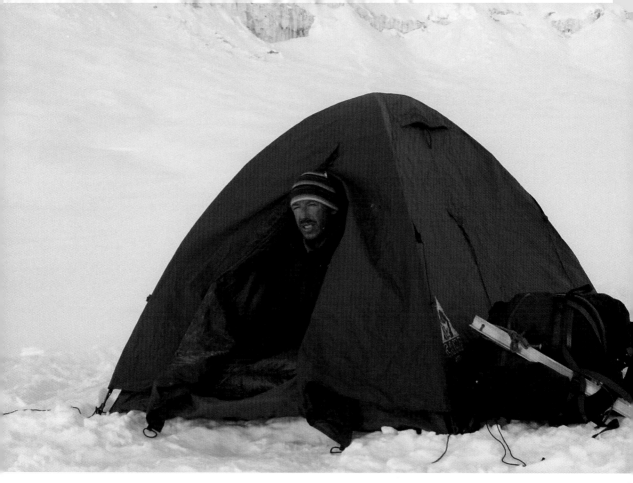

When experiencing mild hypothermia, change your environment or find shelter to escape the cold winds. *Credit: Grant Lipman*

- Replace wet clothing with dry clothing, add wind-resistant and waterproof layers.
- Add insulation under and around the patient.
- Cover head and neck.
- Sweet liquids and food (calories).
- Consider exercise (i.e., calisthenics) to warm up.

Symptoms: HT II – Moderate Hypothermia, 90°F–82°F (32°C–28°C)

- Cessation of shivering at approximately 86°F (30°C).
- Altered level of responsiveness (LOR), lethargic, may appear drunk.
- Combative or irrational.
- Slowed heart and respiratory rates.
- Cannot adequately care for themselves.

Treatment

- Evacuate, as unlikely able to increase core temperature.
- Minimize heat loss and cold exposure with maximum insulation and warm hat.
- Be cautious giving fluids or food because of the risk of vomiting and aspiration.
- If in a coma, handle patient gently as heart is prone to fatal heart rhythms.
- Hypothermia wrap if victim is unable to ambulate.

Symptoms: HT III – Severe Hypothermia, 82°F–75°F (28°C–24°C)

- Comatose with fixed and dilated pupils.
- May have rigid muscles.
- Very slow or absent heart rate.

Treatment

- Handle gently.
- Minimize heat loss and cold exposure with hypothermia wrap.
- Evacuate to a hospital with Intensive Care Unit capabilities.

Symptoms: HT IV – Profound Hypothermia, <75°F (<24°C)

- Likely will appear dead, with very faint or absent vital signs.

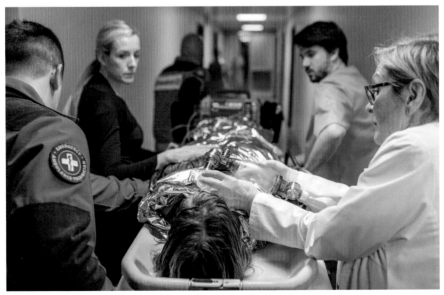

If a patient has profound hypothermia, then it is important to evacuate to a hospital that can adequately treat them.

  SCOUTING GUIDE TO WILDERNESS FIRST AID

Treatment

- Handle gently.
- Minimize heat loss and cold exposure with hypothermia wrap.
- Evacuate to a hospital with Intensive Care Unit capabilities.

Evacuate:

- Mild hypothermia (HT I) that is not able to rewarm.
- Moderate and more severe hypothermia (HT II–IV).

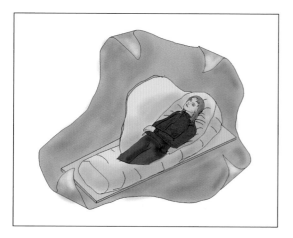
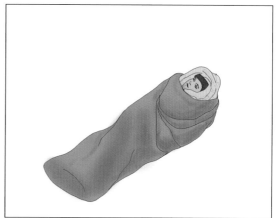

Hypothermia wrap.

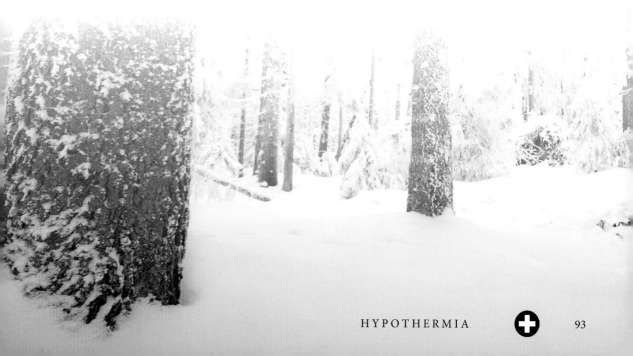

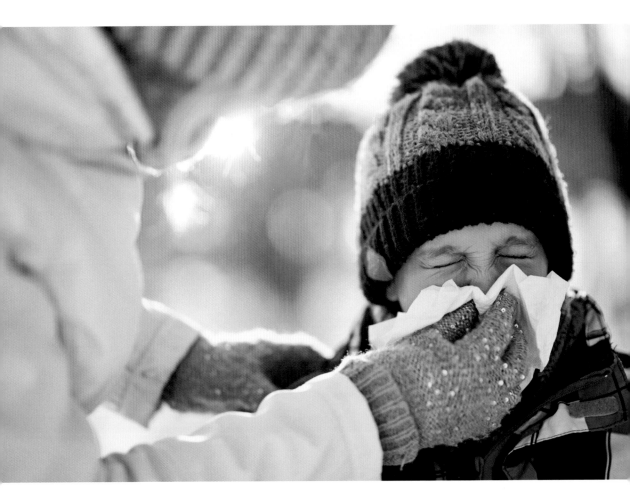

A variety of viral illnesses are common in the wilderness.

CHAPTER 19

INFECTIOUS DISEASE

Travel in wilderness areas around the world will expose travelers to diseases unique to that area. Prior to travel, one should check the Centers for Disease Control and Prevention website (www.cdc.gov) for up-to-date emerging infectious diseases and high risk areas around the world. Being outdoors puts one at risk of exposure to mosquito or tick transmitted diseases such as Lyme disease, Rocky Mountain Spotted Fever, Malaria, and Dengue fever, among others. One should be aware of presenting symptoms and signs of indigenous diseases prior to potential exposure.

Viral "flu-like" illnesses are common in the backcountry and may be responsible for a spectrum of symptoms. While most of these symptoms resolve with time (a few days) and symptomatic care, the course of illness may be prolonged and require rest and an evacuation for complete recuperation. Oftentimes, diseases have a delayed presentation due to an incubation period, and diagnostic workup occurs after a wilderness trip has ended. Ticks that have been attached for less than forty-eight hours have very low rates of Lyme disease transmission.

Ensure good hand hygiene before eating and after using the toilet (to minimize the viral spread and/or self-infecting). Do not ingest untreated water. Do not rinse fruit/vegetables in untreated water. Boil water before drinking.

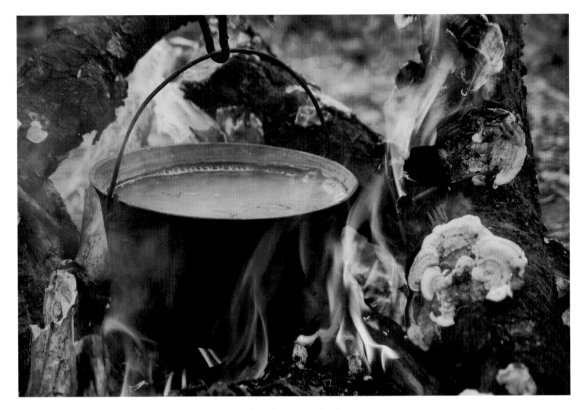

Don't drink untreated water; instead, boil water before use.

Symptoms
- Nausea, vomiting, diarrhea, cough (productive or nonproductive of sputum/mucus), fever, nasal congestion, sore throat, muscle aches, fatigue, headaches.

Treatment
- General management for flu-like illness is treating the symptoms.
- Rest and rehydrate with electrolyte-containing solution. Start slowly (sips every five minutes); then, when the patient is tolerating liquids, aggressively rehydrate with electrolyte-containing fluids.
- Control the nausea with sips of herbal tea, Pepcid and/or Pepto-Bismol as needed (as directed by the instruction label).
- Ibuprofen and acetaminophen for headache, sore throat, muscle aches, per the instructions on the label.
- If frequent diarrhea, Imodium (follow the instructions on the label). Maximum dose is 16mg (eight pills) per day.

- Remove any imbedded ticks with a pair of tweezers, grasping the tick as close to the skin surface as possible. Pull upward gently and with even pressure. Avoid twisting or jerking movements, which can separate tick body or mouth parts which will remain in the skin. Remove any remaining parts, if possible, with tweezers.

Evacuate:

- Fever with headache, stiff neck, and sensitivity to light.
- Flu-like illness with persistent fever and/or difficulty breathing.
- Nausea/vomiting/diarrhea with inability to tolerate fluids for more than twelve hours despite medications.
- A sore throat with inability to swallow water and maintain adequate hydration (feels dizzy on standing and decreased urine output).
- Pale skin, jaundice (yellowed skin), or dark smoky urine.
- High spiking fevers and a non-blanching rash (the rash does not disappear when you press it).

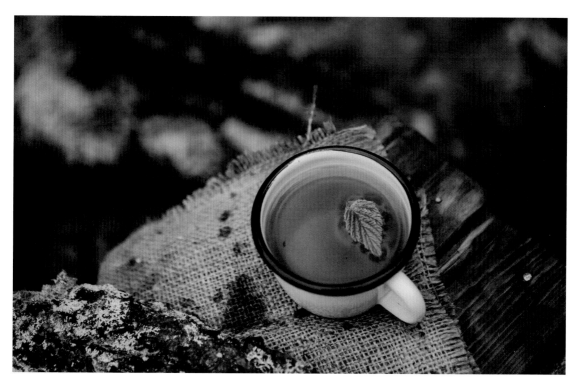

Herbal tea can help manage nausea.

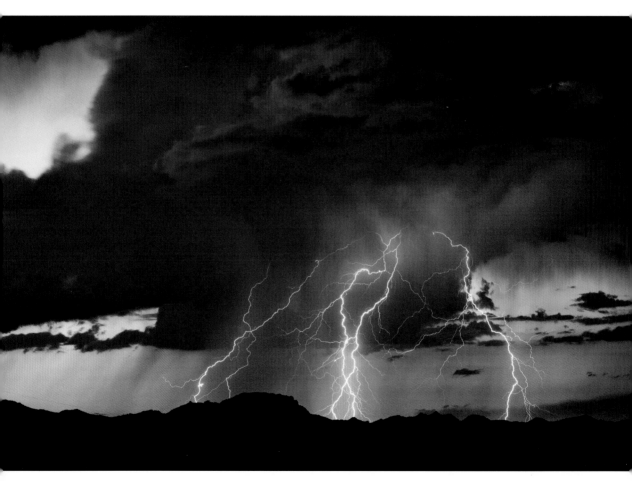

Lightning can be extremely dangerous, so be sure to seek cover.

CHAPTER 20

LIGHTNING

Lightning strikes can affect many organ systems in the body including the heart (fatal rhythm), nervous system (bleeding in the brain, seizures, confusion, amnesia, temporary paralysis), the lungs (respiratory arrest), skin (burns), musculoskeletal system (dislocation or fractures, cold and pulseless extremity from blood vessel spasm), and ears and eyes (deafness or blindness).

The victim of a lightning strike may have fixed and dilated pupils, no breathing, no pulse, and may appear dead. However, the rescuer should immediately perform CPR (*see* **CPR**). While CPR in the wilderness usually has a dismal outcome, the massive amount of energy contained in a lightning strike may short circuit the breathing center of the brain and the normal beating rhythm of the heart. While the heart has inherent automaticity and will usually restart spontaneously, the lungs do not have this same ability. Unfortunately the lack of oxygen in this situation will eventually cause the heart to stop beating and the victim will die. So frequent pulse checks during CPR may reveal a heartbeat that has regained a healthy rhythm, but they may need continued assistance with rescue breaths for five or ten minutes until the stunned respiratory center of the brain gets back on-line.

Lightning can strike an individual directly, harm through a concussive blast (from exploding air), or cause injury through side splash (where the lightning jumps from its target to the victim) or through ground current (radiation of the electrical charge through the ground)

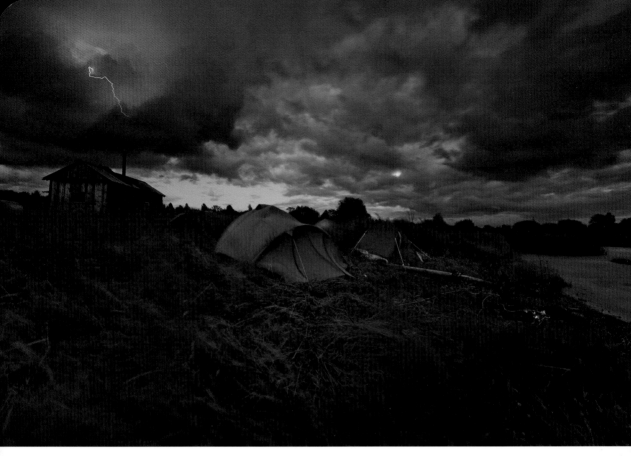

Small shelters like tents are an inadequate shelter during lightning storms.

and conduction. The best treatment is prevention, and awareness of high risk topography, situations, and safest locations can minimize risk.

Lightning Prevention

- If time between lightning and thunder is thirty seconds or less, people are in danger of a strike and should seek appropriate cover.
- Wait at least thirty minutes after lightning/thunder before resuming outdoor activity.
- Seek shelter: big buildings, deep caves (three times deeper than wide), metal vehicles.
- Avoid small shelters (e.g., tents), peaks, overhangs, and gullies that may increase risk of ground current injury.
- Avoid contact with metal objects and objects taller than you.
- Do not stand near isolated tall trees (which can injure through side splash).

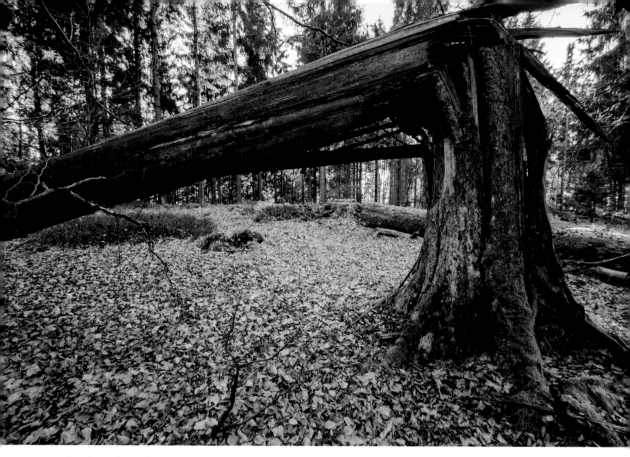

Avoid tall, isolated trees that could fall and injure you during a storm.

- Seek a low area near groups of small trees—*not* a clearing where a person may be the tallest object.
- If you are in the open, sit down in a lightning crouch with the legs together to theoretically minimize the voltage difference.
- Sit on nonconductive padding (pack, pad, rope, lifejacket).
- If in a group, spread out more than one hundred feet between individuals if

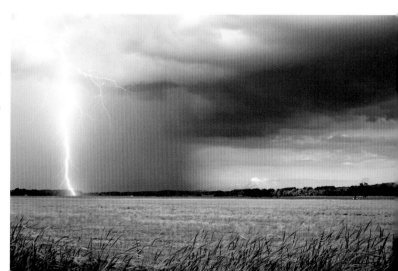

During lightning storms, avoid being in a clearing or an area where you could be the tallest object.

possible, while maintaining visual contact (making sure that trip leaders are spread out as well).

- Get out of the water.
- Keep in mind that lightning can strike the same spot twice.
- Lightning in the mountains is more likely in the afternoons.

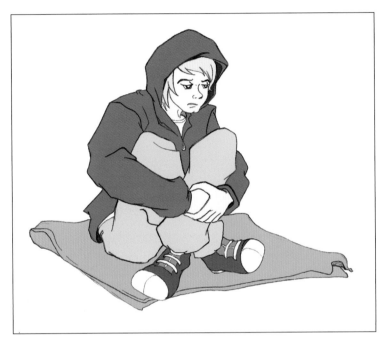

Lightning crouch.

Treatment

- Perform CPR if no pulse. Continue until spontaneously breathing or the rescuer is exhausted.
- If multiple victims require CPR, those with lightning burns to the head have lower rates of survival due to potential devastating brain bleeds.
- Treat injuries as needed.
- Aggressive hydration.

Evacuate: Any patient struck by lightning, with a lightning burn or injury, or unconscious or change in LOR after nearby lightning.

CHAPTER 21

LUNG PROBLEMS

There can be many causes for shortness of breath, ranging from minor and non-life threatening issues like anxiety with hyperventilation, to viral infections and inflammatory diseases like bronchitis, to a serious bacterial pneumonia that needs antibiotics, or a medical emergency like a collapsed lung or blood clot. A thorough history will help differentiate the severity of the underlying cause and likely indicate whether an evacuation is necessary.

An infection of the airways or lung tissue is usually from a virus or bacteria. These can both cause high fevers, persistent coughing, phlegm production, and shortness of breath. Treat the fever with Tylenol or Motrin and encourage drinking to combat dehydration. Viral infections often present with associated runny nose, sore throat, muscular aches, and pain. That being said, viruses suppress the immune system, which potentially allows a bacterial infection to worsen. So be suspicious for a secondary infection when someone recovering from a viral syndrome suddenly relapses with a high fever and worsening cough.

A collapsed lung (pneumothorax) can occur from blunt chest trauma or spontaneously in a young healthy person when air escapes from a lung cell, and gets trapped between the chest wall and the lung. The chest pain is sudden, severe, and sharp, and may lead to guarded shallow breaths with shortness of breath. It can be difficult to discern the difference in decreased breath sounds over the area of pain. But if symptoms are worsening or severe, the person should be evacuated. Alternatively, similar symptoms with reproducible tenderness when the chest wall is pushed upon may be a viral infection of the rib lining (costochondritis).

This is not associated with shortness of breath, is not serious, and can be treated with Motrin as directed by the instruction label (every six to eight hours as needed).

Similar symptoms as a pneumothorax but more insidious is a blood clot in the lungs (pulmonary embolus). The pain may be dull or sharp, often worse on inspiration, can be increased when lying flat, and associated with shortness of breath, rapid heart rate at rest, and sometimes fever. Pulmonary embolisms are a great mimic for almost any other disease process in the lungs, and risk factors include: birth control, recent prolonged immobility, cancer, and pregnancy, Diagnosis and treatment are only available in a hospital.

Symptoms

- Rapid breathing rate.
- History of asthma or chronic lung disease.
- Audible wheezes.
- Numbness/tingling in the hands and feet.
- Worsening shortness of breath with exertion.
- Chest pain associated with shortness of breath.
- Anxiety.
- Fever and cough with sputum.

⚠ **Red Flags:** Shortness of breath on exertion, or with chest pain. Cough with shortness of breath and/or fever.

Treatment: Anxiety

- If the patient appears anxious with rapid rate of breathing, tingling in hands/feet (suspected anxiety attack), and no history of asthma—calm patient by being direct and reassuring.
- Give sack to breathe into.

Treatment: Wheeze

Giving the patient a bag to breathe into can help steady their breathing.

- If there is a history of asthma, assist patient with their own medicines (inhaler).
- **Severe:** Gasping with three- to five-word sentences, sweating, may appear fatigued or sleepy. Above medicines and EpiPen to outside of upper thigh. May repeat in five to twenty minutes if initial dose is ineffective or there is a recurrence of symptoms.

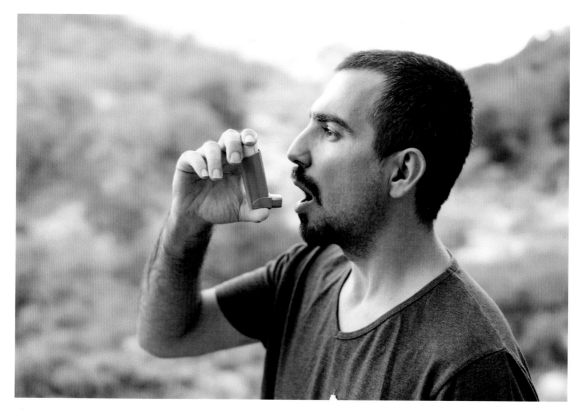

If the patient has an inhaler, using it can help relieve their wheezing.

Treatment: Fever

- Cough with sputum, fever, and worsening shortness of breath, exacerbated by exertion—suspect pneumonia.

Treatment: Chest Pain

- Shortness of breath with chest pain, may be sharp, worse on inhalation, and not reproducible.

Evacuate:

- Asthma attack not responding to the person's inhaler or requiring EpiPen.
- Asthma that does not resolve or worsens despite appropriate medication.
- Cough with fever and worsening shortness of breath.
- Shortness of breath associated with chest pain.
- Shortness of breath that worsens with exertion.

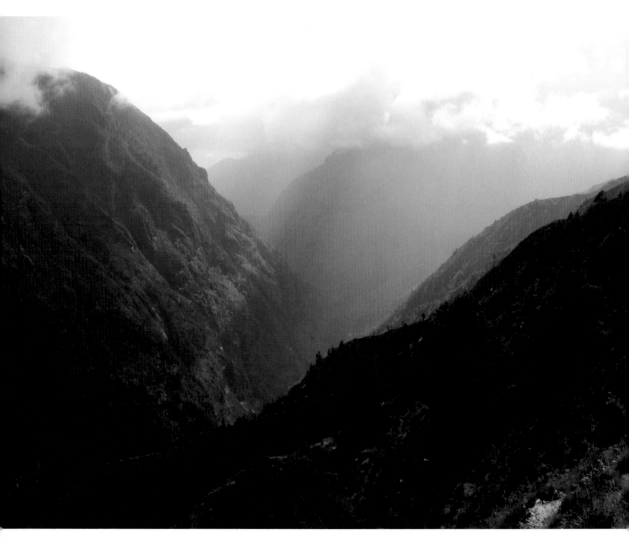

CHAPTER 22
MALE GENITAL PROBLEMS

Testicular pain after trauma is the most likely cause of male genital pain in the wilderness—where the severity of pain dictates your ability to manage the situation. If a testicle suddenly becomes painful it may be due to its rotation and twisting on the cord that supplies blood to the scrotum (torsion). This is a surgical emergency and may lead to death of the testicle. If the pain is severe and unrelenting, "detorting" the testicle may resolve the situation while arranging evacuation for definitive care. Some testicular pain can be from an infection. While infectious problems as well as surgical issues will be a challenge to differentiate, delay can result in loss of viability of the testicle so the decision to evacuate for definitive care should err on the conservative side.

Symptoms
- Testicular pain, often one-sided.
- Pain relieved by elevation of the testes
- Hurts to walk or lie flat.

⚠ **Red Flag:** Spontaneous severe testicular pain.

Treatment
- Pain management with Motrin (follow the instructions on the label).
- Cool compress.

- Elevation and support of the testicles.
- Detorting a testes involves grasping it gently and rotating it outwards, like opening a book page. If this worsens the pain, return the teste to its original lie.

Evacuate: Any patient with severe testicular pain.

SCOUTING GUIDE TO WILDERNESS FIRST AID

CHAPTER 23

MUSCULOSKELETAL INJURIES

The severity and need for evacuation of a musculoskeletal injury in the wilderness setting will likely be dictated by the ability to use that extremity. For example, a twisted ankle that is too painful to walk on may require a similar treatment of immobilization in the field and subsequent evacuation as a broken ankle. If the injury is a direct blow or fall, always consider a broken bone. If the injury is from a twisting motion, a sprain or strain is most common. A sprain and strain are injuries to the rubber band–like connective tissues (ligaments and tendons) attaching the bones and muscles to each other. Depending on the severity of the tear to these tissues, there may be bruising, swelling, or joint instability. Look at the uninjured extremity to compare deformity, angulation, and overall appearance. Immobilization of the injured area will decrease pain by limiting movement.

Sometimes overuse of an extremity can lead to inflammation, swelling, and pain without an acute injury. The pain and swelling from an overuse injury can be severe, and while usually not serious can potentially be debilitating. For example, a snow shoeing trip with severe Achilles tendinitis would be miserable. Likewise, forearm tendonitis or shoulder or elbow bursitis while canoeing could end the activity. An anti-inflammatory like Motrin and rest can improve the pain.

Dislocations result in an oddly shaped joint that cannot be normally ranged. The most common dislocations are the shoulder, finger, ankle, and patella (knee cap). Any dislocations may be associated with a broken bone. Consider reducing a dislocation in the field if you

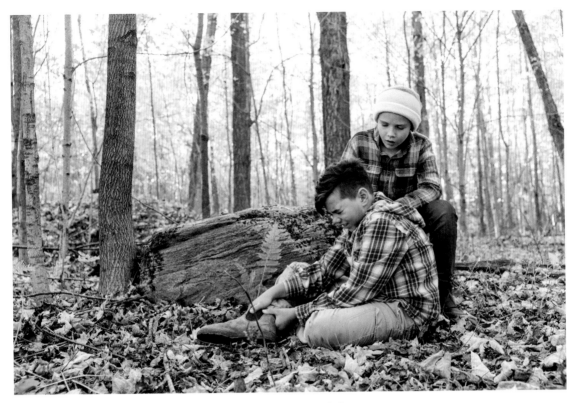

A twisted ankle can be severe enough to limit mobility.

have specific training in the technique and if the patient is amenable to an attempt. In general, both the difficulty of reduction and the amount of long-term complications increase with delay in reduction attempts. Always check CSM—**circulation** (healthy pinking of the nail bed after pressure should take less than three seconds), **sensation** (dull versus sharp differentiation), and **movement** of the joint—and note the status and any change after the reduction attempt. All dislocation/reduction attempts should be performed with a calm and reassuring voice, applying slow, gentle, and constant effort. Avoid sudden jerky movements which can increase the individual's pain, and decrease both the ability to overcome resistant muscle spasm as well as the victim's willingness to allow a second attempt if initially unsuccessful. If pain or resistance, go slower (think of the reduction movement like a minute hand on a clock, rather than the second hand), while maintaining constant force and calming voice.

Symptoms: Broken Bone

- Angulation or movement where no joint exists ("a false joint").

SCOUTING GUIDE TO WILDERNESS FIRST AID

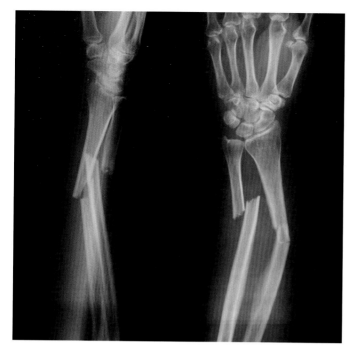

X-ray of a broken arm.

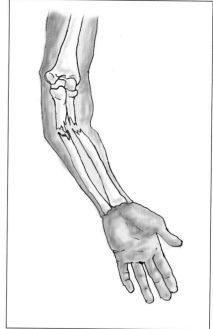

Angulation.

- Point tenderness on the bone.
- Inability to bear weight.
- Hear or feel the grinding of bones together.
- Swelling or discoloration at the point of pain.

⚠ **Red Flags:** Loss of CSM, angulation, or severe tenderness to a bony point.

Treatment

- Remove jewelry.
- Pad bony points with soft material.
- If weight bearing/usable, suspect a sprain/strain and apply compressive bandage wrap.
- If not weight bearing or patient is unable to use extremity, suspect broken bone and apply sling or rigid splint (SAM splint).
- Sling/Splint: Immobilize joint above and below injured site in natural position.
  - ➤ **Wrist:** Splint in position like holding a beverage can (SAM splint).
  - ➤ **Ankle/Elbow:** Splint in 90-degree flexion (SAM splint/sling/sleeping pad). Secure firmly but not tightly.
  - ➤ **Collarbone:** Immobilize the affected extremity with a sling, and may further

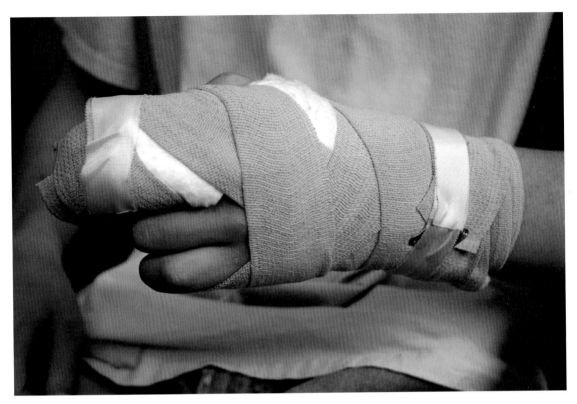

Broken fingers can be taped together.

minimize movement and pain with a swathe (a circumferential bandage around both the upper arm and the trunk).

> **Fingers:** Broken fingers can be buddy taped together.
> **Rib fractures:** Wrap a compression wrap or similar wide bandage circumferentially around the fractured ribs to effectively buddy tape them to the uninjured neighboring ribs. Encourage the person to take deep breaths to minimize collapse of compressed lung tissue and subsequent infection.
> **Lower leg:** Rigid splint on either side, or behind the injured area. A sleeping bag can be wrapped around the injured part like a burrito and secured with tape. Make sure to put padding in the fossa behind the knee.

- Motrin or Tylenol as needed, and per the instruction labels.
- Check CSM before and after splint application.
- If open bone, irrigate copiously with drinkable water, then cover with antibiotic ointment and sterile/clean gauze.

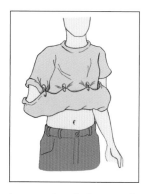
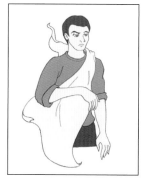
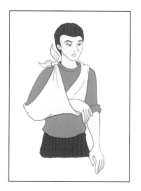
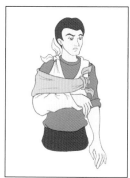

Improvised sling with safety pins.

Sling from fabric or triangular gauze.

Symptoms: Shoulder Dislocation

- Loss of natural curve of shoulder (shoulder appears squared).
- Holding affected arm up and away from body.
- Unable to touch unaffected (opposite) shoulder with the fingers of the injured arm.

Note: Only attempt reductions if trained in the procedure *and* patient is amenable.

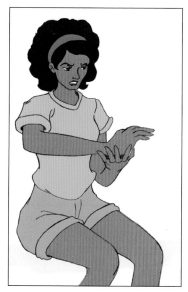
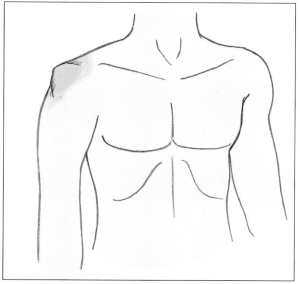

Body position of a dislocated shoulder.

Appearance of dislocated shoulder.

Treatment

- Remove jewelry.

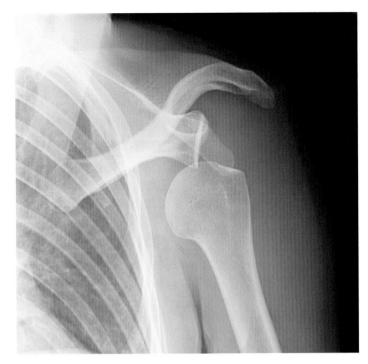

X-ray of a dislocated shoulder.

- Assess CSM.
- Reduce dislocation.
- If successful reduction, you may feel or hear a "thunk" and significant resolution of the individual's pain.
- Recheck CSM and sling arm.

Knee-Wrap Self-Reduction Technique:

- Sit the injured person down with bent knees.
- Clasp both their hands around knees and have them lean back, *slowly* inducing constant traction to overcome the shoulder muscle spasm until the shoulder reduces.

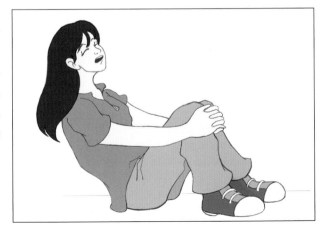

Shoulder reduction by knee-wrap technique.

SCOUTING GUIDE TO WILDERNESS FIRST AID

Tree-Hug Reduction Technique:

- Have the injured person wrap their arms around a slender tree (hugging it).
- Clasp both their hands around trunk and have them lean back, *slowly*, putting all their body weight into it, until the constant traction overcomes the shoulder's muscle spasm and the shoulder reduces.

Spaso Reduction Technique:

- Have the injured person lie on his back, relaxing the shoulder to allow the shoulder blade to rest on the ground, and with calm and gentle voice and movements, grasp the injured arm by the wrist, holding straight up (perpendicular to the body).
- Apply gentle vertical traction for a few minutes while holding the arm straight.
- Keep patient relaxed while doing this, so the shoulder blade stays flat and in contact with the ground.
- Apply gentle external rotation (rotate toward the thumb side of the hand).
- After a few minutes of traction, reduction should occur.

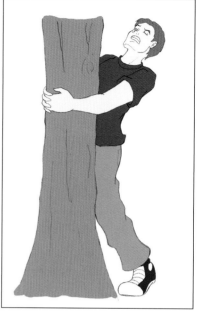

Shoulder reduction by tree-hug technique.

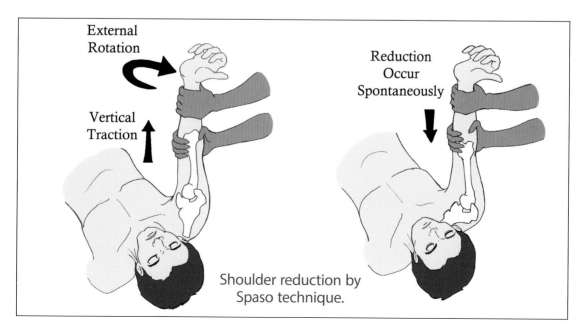

Shoulder reduction by Spaso technique.

External Rotation Technique*:

- Have injured person lie on his or her back, and with calm and gentle voice and movements, have them bend their affected elbow at 90 degrees.
- Holding affected arm above and at the elbow, bend the shoulder to 90 degrees, which will slowly bring the arm out and away from body.
- Angle the point of the elbow towards the rib cage (which will tilt the arm upwards and outwards).
- Rotate arm outward like opening a book (so back of hand and forearm are facing the ground).
- If necessary, from the open book position, you can bring the arm up (to end up in a position similar to an overhand throw), at which point reduction should occur.
- Be patient, as this process may take five to ten minutes. If resistance is met or pain increases, slow or stop movement, holding position until pain is overcome.

* This technique can be performed with the injured person sitting upright with a straight back, ideally against a vertical support.

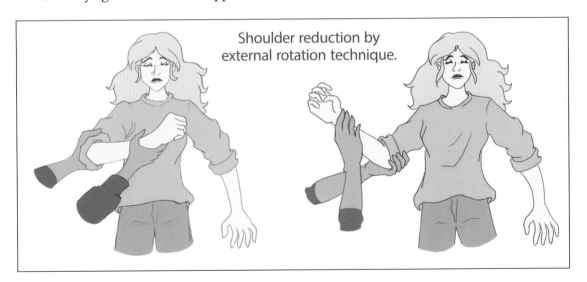

Shoulder reduction by external rotation technique.

Symptoms: Kneecap Dislocation

- Knee feels unstable/leg collapsed.
- Kneecap is repositioned to the outer aspect of the leg.

Treatment

- Sit patient up, flexed at hip, making a 90-degree angle with the leg and torso.
- Straighten leg while pushing kneecap toward the midline (with continuous rapid motion).
- Hyperextend leg (bend the knee opposite of natural joint movement). Knee cap should pop back in.
- Post-reduction patient can weight bear and walk out.
- Immobilize knee with sleeping pad/rigid splint (fashion "suspenders" to keep pad from slipping if needed).

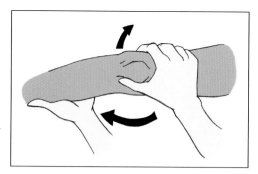

Kneecap reduction.

Symptoms: Finger or Toe Dislocation

- Fingers angulated at a joint.
- Unable to bend finger joint.

Treatment

- Slow steady movement.
- Do not jerk.
- Holding the injured digit partially flexed, pull on the end towards the angle of the dislocation (pull the direction the finger or toe is pointing in).
- Pull until you hear a "pop" and joint appears to have normal orientation.
- Buddy-tape finger or toe (with adjacent finger or toe).

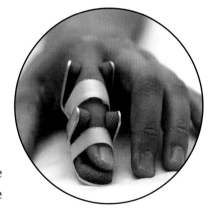

Use a splint to immobilize and splint the finger or toe dislocation.

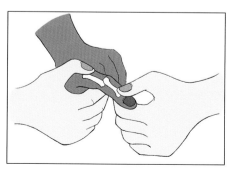

(Left) Finger reduction.

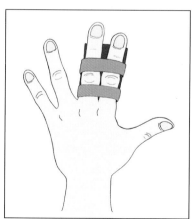

(Right) Finger buddy-taping.

Symptoms: Ankle Dislocation

- Angulation (often pointing outwards from midline).
- Bony protrusion/tenting of skin.
- Pain and inability to weight bear.

Treatment

- Have the injured person lie down with affected leg bent at the knee.
- Have one person hold and stabilize the lower leg at the calf (for counter-traction, providing an anchor).
- Have the second person grasp mid-foot just below the ball of the foot (one hand) and at the heel (second hand).
- Applying constant strong force, pull away from body in direction foot is pointing (traction).
- Once a release of tension is felt, guide foot back to midline.
- Check CSM and splint.

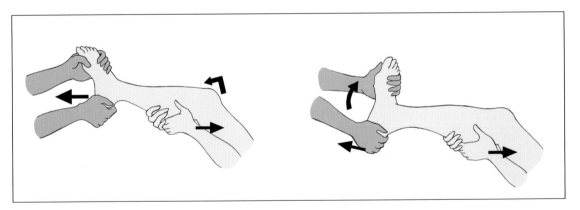

Ankle reduction technique.

🚁 Evacuate:

- Any patient with an unreduced dislocation.
- Any patient with altered CSM before or after reduction.
- Any *unusable* musculoskeletal injury, whether a suspected sprain, strain, broken bone, or dislocation. Either due to pain or joint instability.

  SCOUTING GUIDE TO WILDERNESS FIRST AID

CHAPTER 24

NERVOUS SYSTEM

Injury to the brain from a blood clot or bleeding in a vessel can present as many different symptoms, depending on the area and amount of tissue involved. Strokes can cause symptoms (neurologic deficit) that impair speech, vision, motor function, sensation, balance or coordination, level of consciousness, of even the ability to breathe. Strokes are sudden, with weakness or numbness that typically involve one side of the body, can be either transient or constant, and may be associated with a severe "thunderclap" headache.

Patients with known seizure disorder (epilepsy) are usually on prescription medicine to control their seizures. Ideally, they should have their seizures well controlled by medicine or be seizure free for at least six months, carry their own medicine, and be cleared by their medical doctor before embarking into the wilderness. Seizures can occur as a primary disorder (i.e., epilepsy) or secondary to an environmental injury or other illness (e.g., low blood sugar, low salt level, heat stroke, head trauma, stroke, etc.). If the patient does not have a known diagnosis of epilepsy, look for potentially reversible causes.

Symptoms: Neurologic Deficit
- Decrease in muscle strength or sensation on one side (face, arm, and/or leg).
- Unsteady gait.
- Dizziness.
- One-sided facial droop.

- Severe thunderclap headache.
- Bilateral leg weakness/numbness progressing up the body.

Red Flags: Any neurologic deficit or change in level of responsiveness (LOR).

Treatment
- Place the patient in a position of comfort unless unconscious, then position patient in the recovery position.
- Thorough physical exam to document neurologic deficits and any changes.

Symptoms: Seizure
- Patient feels encroaching seizure (aura).
- Blank staring gaze for few seconds.
- Involuntary movement of a localized extremity without loss of consciousness.
- Generalized shaking of entire body with unconsciousness.
- Incontinence of bowel/bladder.
- Altered level of responsiveness (LOR) post-seizure.

⚠ **Red Flags:** Any seizure in a person without known epilepsy (first-time seizure). Multiple seizures or prolonged duration than usual.

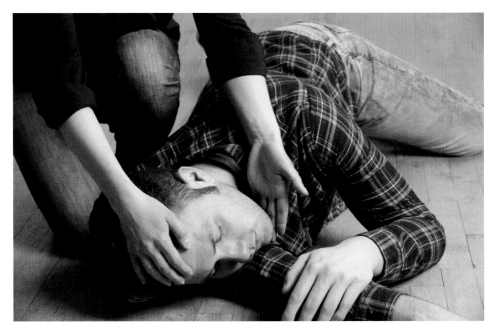

After a patient stops seizing, move them into recovery position.

✚ SCOUTING GUIDE TO WILDERNESS FIRST AID

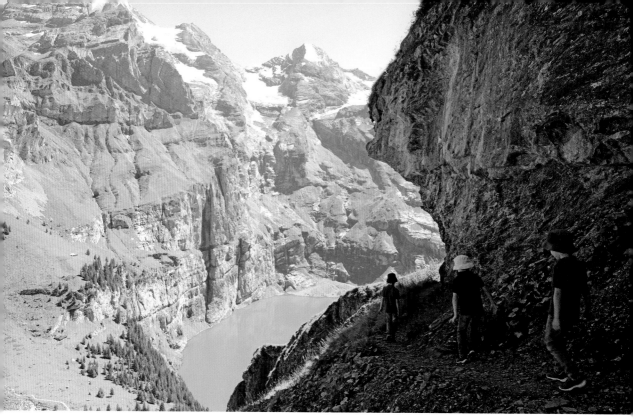

If an epileptic patient just recovered from a seize, do not bring them into hazardous terrain, such as narrow cliffs.

Treatment

- Protect patient (move patient away from environmental hazards).
- Place pad under head if generalized seizure.
- If patient appears to be choking or turns blue, use head tilt/jaw thrust maneuver to open airway. Never put your finger or another object in a seizing person's mouth.
- Once recovered, position patient in recovery position.
- Perform complete physical exam to check for injuries.

Evacuate:
- Any patient with a focal neurologic deficit.
- Any new seizure.
- Patient with epilepsy, who has multiple seizures without regaining consciousness, or a prolonged seizure over fifteen minutes.
- Any epileptic on trip who has had a simple seizure and is now going into potentially hazardous terrain (e.g., narrow cliff hike, kayaking, etc.).
- Any patient with an altered level of responsiveness (LOR) of unknown origin.

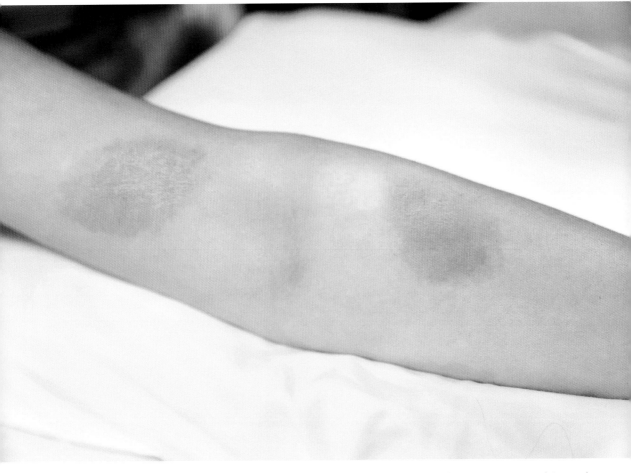

Stinging nettle can cause a skin rash.

CHAPTER 25
SKIN IRRITATION

The skin can be irritated from a resin (urushiol) found in the sap of certain plants. The most common toxic plants are poison oak, poison ivy, stinging nettles, and poison sumac that causes a toxic reaction to the skin (contact dermatitis). Poison ivy can appear as a shrub, or grow to a tree size with reddish leaves when young or dark red green leaves when older. Like poison oak, remember, "leaves of three, let it be." Post-exposure, a thorough washing of the exposed skin with soap and water is necessary to remove the resin, as it is irreversibly bound to the skin within thirty to sixty minutes. Individuals have different sensitivities to urushiol, with a reaction that can occur within eight hours to as long as three weeks. The resin can be spread on clothing, camping equipment, or the fur of pets; and last for years if not washed off. Red, swollen, and irritated skin with lines of small blisters are the classic presentation. The blister fluid is not contagious, and the body's immune reaction can cause rash and blisters on parts of the skin that were not exposed. Inhaled smoke from burning plants can also cause a reaction to the nose, mouth, and throat.

A bacterial infection of the skin (cellulitis) presents as spreading redness, warmth, pain, and may have collections of pus (abscess). The redness can be raised, swollen, and confluent, or linear streaks. There may

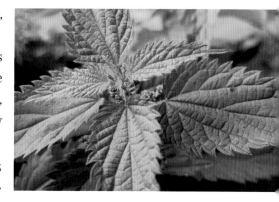

Learn to identify toxic plants such as poison oak.

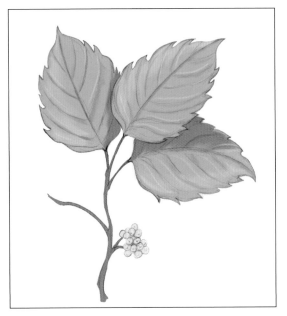

Poison ivy.

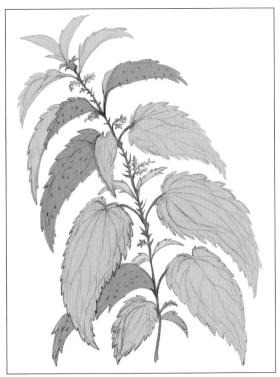

Poison oak.

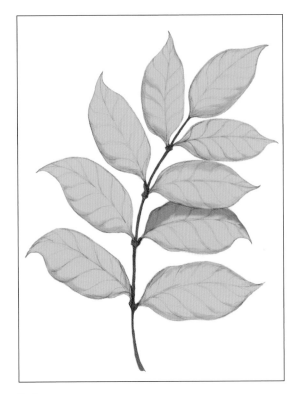

Poison sumac.

Stinging nettle.

  SCOUTING GUIDE TO WILDERNESS FIRST AID

be an associated fever. Any concerning signs of a bacterial infection will require evacuation for medical evaluation and antibiotics.

Symptoms

- Itchy red rash, fluid-filled blisters. Skin irritation may be delayed for up to three weeks.

Treatment

- Wash the affected area (or suspected exposed area) well with soap and water, ideally within thirty minutes of exposure.
- Wash all clothes and equipment that may have been exposed.
- Once the rash appears, itching can be relieved with hydrocortisone cream. More severe itching can be treated with oral Benadryl (follow the instructions on the label).
- Severe blistering may need a two-week prescription steroid (prednisone).

Evacuate:

- Any reaction that involves the eyes, genitals, airway, or breathing.
- Skin irritation that is too uncomfortable to continue trip.
- Any signs of infection to skin (e.g., spreading redness, warmth, and/or pus).

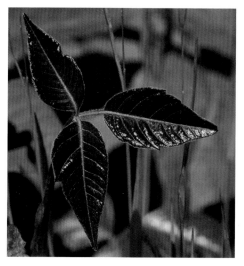

Poison ivy.

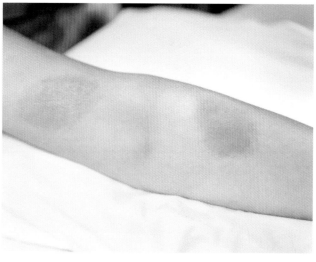

A rash caused by poison ivy or other toxic plants can be relieved with Hydrocortisone cream.

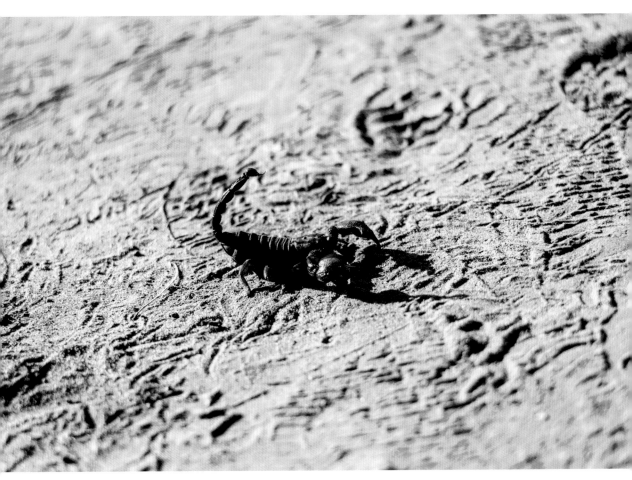

A bark scorpion. All scorpion stings are cause for immediate evacuation.

CHAPTER 26

TOXINS, BITES, AND STINGS

The effects of a toxin from a bite or sting from an animal or insect can range from a mild local reaction to a critical life-threatening situation. The most concerning toxin in North America is from a snakebite. There are two types of venomous indigenous snakes, the pit vipers (e.g., rattlesnakes, water moccasins, copperheads) and coral snakes. Most injuries are from pit vipers. Approximately 25 percent of pit viper bites are "dry bites," and do not result in envenomation. However, as symptoms and signs of envenomation may be delayed for up to six to eight hours, and the definitive treatment is antivenin, all snakebites should be evacuated for observation in a hospital setting. If the victim is more than a few hours from a hospital, walking the person out on their own (at the risk of increasing circulation of the toxin) may be more expeditious to decrease the time getting to antivenin, than going for a rescue.

Typical signs of a pit viper envenomation are severe burning pain at the bite site (two puncture wounds), swelling and bruising around the bite area that spreads towards the center of the body, difficulty breathing and rapid heart rate, weakness, and collapse. Fatalities within minutes of a snakebite is very rare, and usually due to anaphylaxis (*see* **Allergic Reaction**). Most coral snakes are found in the Southeast or Southwest United States. These have a neurotoxin, which have a rapid onset and present with numbness, weakness, vomiting, drooling, slurred speech, difficulty breathing, altered level of responsiveness (LOR), and collapse.

If Bitten by a Snake:

- Do NOT panic. Calm down the victim, offer reassurance, and plan the evacuation.
- Avoid further injuries. Most snakebites are defensive strikes, so keeping a distance of at least the length of the snake should be safe.
- Attempt to identify the snake with a picture. Do NOT attempt to capture the snake as that may result in an additional victim.
- Do NOT place a tourniquet. This could cause further tissue damage to the underlying skin and muscle already made fragile from the destructive toxins.
- Place a splint to immobilize the extremity if not using that extremity to self-evacuate.
- Do NOT place ice on a wound.
- Do NOT apply a Sawyer extractor pump (they don't help, they just suck).
- If bitten by a coral snake and trained in the application, use the pressure-immobilization technique.

The black widow spider found in North America has a bite that can cause significant injury. The female black widow is a glossy black with a red dot or hourglass shape on its back. Its bite is felt like a pinprick, and severe painful muscle spasms usually begin within the hour and can progress in intensity and include vomiting and difficulty breathing. It may be more severe for a pregnant woman or child. Symptoms are treated with pain medicine and usually resolve within one to two days. There is an anti-venom reserved for severe envenomations.

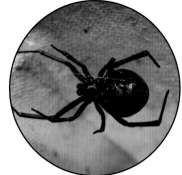

A black widow spider. *Credit: Shenrich91, CC BY-SA 3.0*

In North America, the one scorpion which has a dangerous sting is the bark scorpion (see image on page 126), found in the dry desert habitats of the Southwest. This small yellowish-brown scorpion has a sting that causes immediate burning pain, which is exacerbated by tapping on the site. There is potential for progression of systemic and neurologic symptoms including: sweating, drooling, muscle spasms, seizures, and breathing difficulties and collapse. As symptoms are progressive and may require intensive care unit medical support, all scorpion stings should be evacuated.

Ingested plants and berries found in the wilderness may cause dangerous toxicities. Similar to overdoses of drugs or medicines, the inciting agent may be difficult to identify. Regardless, the goals of treatment are the same: minimize exposure, dilute (if possible), and maximize excretion of the toxin. Give symptomatic support, as specific antidotes are unlikely to be available in a wilderness environment.

Symptoms: Snakebite
- Oozing at site, significant pain from bite, swelling, bruising, discoloration.
- Possible shortness of breath, wheezing.
- Possible numbness to mouth or tongue, muscle weakness, collapse.

⚠ **Red Flags:** Any swelling or skin discoloration, severe persistent pain at bite site, or any neurologic symptoms indicates envenomation.

Treatment
- Remove constricting clothing and jewelry.
- Clean area and dress wound with antibiotic ointment.
- Mark site of initial bruising/swelling by circling with a pen.
- If difficulty breathing/wheeze, treat like anaphylaxis (*see* **Severe** in the **Allergic Reaction** section).
- Evacuate all victims of snakebites.

🚁 **Evacuate:**
- All snakebites, regardless of swelling or bruising, as symptoms may progress over the next six to eight hours.
- Ambulate if able (as minimal time to an emergency room is the most important consideration), otherwise send for assistance.

Symptoms: Spider Bite
- Pin prick or painless bite.
- Severe muscle cramps and pain in bitten extremity.
- May involve stomach or chest muscles, vomiting, difficulty breathing, blistering or redness to site.

Treatment
- Clean bite with soap and water.
- Ibuprofen or Tylenol as needed for pain, per the instructions on the labels.
- Apply cold compress to area.

🚁 **Evacuate:**
- Severe pain within sixty minutes of bite.

- Any systemic symptoms.
- Any black widow spider bite.

Symptoms: Scorpion Sting

- Painful sting, burning pain to site, numbness to site, positive "tap test," paralysis, muscle spasms, blurred vision, difficulty swallowing, slurred speech. breathing problems.

Treatment

- Apply cool compress to site.
- Ibuprofen or Tylenol as needed for pain, per the instructions on the label.
- **Evacuate:** All scorpion stings. Symptoms may progress over six to eight hours. Evacuate early.

Symptoms: Ingested Toxin

- Mild nausea, vomiting, diarrhea, headache, collapse, seizures.

Treatment

- Remove patient from offending toxin (i.e., tent with stove possibly causing carbon monoxide toxicity).
- Treat nausea and vomiting with sips of herbal tea and Pepcid (as directed by instruction label).
- If absorbed toxin, wash off area with soap and water.
- If able, contact the American Association of Poison Control Centers (1-800-222-1222).
- **Evacuate:**
  - Inability to tolerate fluids.
  - Persistent weakness due to vomiting.
  - Collapse.

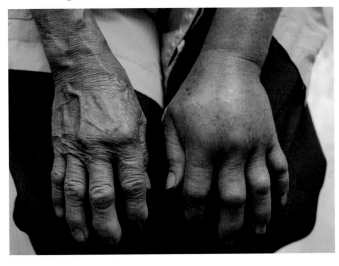

Swelling or bruising at the site of a snakebite is a red flag and cause for evacuation.

Symptoms: Stings or Bites (Insects, Bees, Wasps, Ants, Ticks)

- Local pain, swelling, redness, weakness, nausea, vomiting, fever.
- Allergic reaction.

Treatment

- Scrape off stinger.
- If tick is imbedded, grab the head with tweezers as near to the skin as possible, and with constant gentle force, pull up and away.
- Wash area well with soap and water.
- Cold compress to area.
- Benadryl (as directed by the instruction label) for local inflammation/itching (*see* **Allergic Reaction**).
- If wheezing or difficulty breathing, treat for anaphylaxis.

Evacuate: Any sting with associated breathing difficulties or severe allergic reaction/anaphylaxis.

Symptoms: Jellyfish

- Skin irritation, severe burning, itching, nausea and vomiting, headache, muscle aches, dizziness, numbness, seizure, collapse, altered level of responsiveness (LOR).

Treatment

- Rinse wound with sea water (avoid fresh water).
- Rinse with vinegar (avoid vinegar if suspected Portuguese man-of-war).
- Make a paste of sand and water; scrape off extra stinging cells with edge of card/knife.

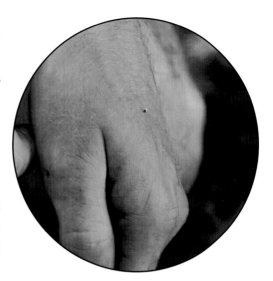

If stung by an insect, begin treatment by removing the stinger.

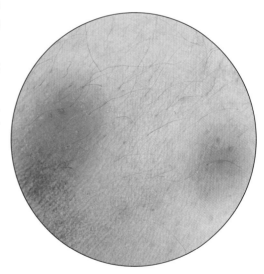

Taking Benadryl can help reduce the inflammation and itching from a bug bite.

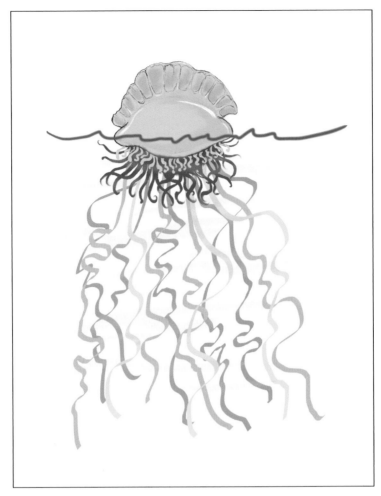

Portuguese man-of-war jellyfish.

- Apply hot water after stinging cells have been scraped off.
- If allergic reaction or anaphylaxis, treat accordingly.

Evacuate: Severe pain, any severe allergic reaction, or any breathing problems or neurologic problems.

CHAPTER 27

TRAUMA

The first premise in evaluating any trauma victim is to ensure that the scene is safe for the rescuer; otherwise good intentioned assistance may lead to a second victim. Rock fall, animal attack, thin ice, or a fast river, for example, must all be taken into consideration *prior* to approaching a hurt individual. Always consider the mechanism of injury (MOI) that may have injured the spine, and if concerning, the hurt individual should be kept still with the rescuer's hands while evaluating potential injuries. Damage to the spinal cord can cause permanent paralysis or death. Damage to the bones in the neck (cervical spine) can paralyze the body's ability to breathe. So proper care and management of the suspected spinal injury may prevent an injury to the bones around the spinal cord damaging the underlying nerves.

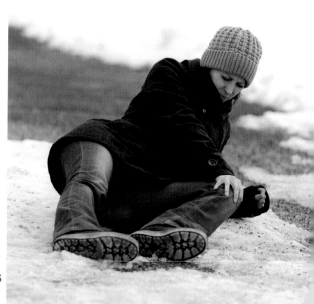

Considering the mechanism of injury—such as slipping on ice—can increase awareness of a potential spinal cord injury and avoid further damage.

Trauma Best Practices

- Take *early* spinal precautions with patients prior to the **Focused Assessment of Cervical Spine (FACS).**
- Always ensure good breathing and a clear airway first.
- If a second rescuer is available, have them hold the cervical spine stable.
- Assume there is a spinal injury if a patient has altered level of responsiveness (LOR) or is unconscious.
- If it's necessary to roll a person (log roll) or move them to a safer environment, the movement should be coordinated by the rescuer at the head, ensuring the rolling/moving is done as a unit with as little angulation or side-to-side movement as possible.
- Ask the victim if there is any spine or back midline pain, weakness, or numbness to hands or feet prior to examination.
- Feel along the entire spine, looking for midline tenderness.
- If the person is conscious and reliable, the utilization of the **FACS** can determine the presence or absence of a bony injury that could cause spinal cord compromise.
- If there is any suspicion for cervical spinal injury, err on the side of caution with full immobilization and then necessary evacuation.

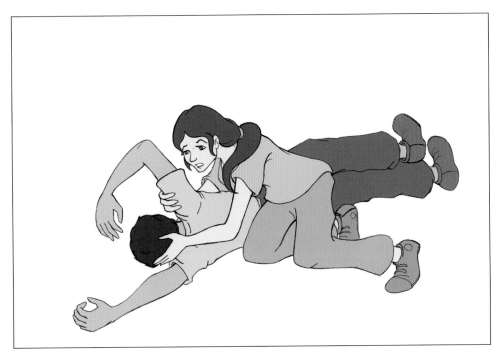

One-person log roll.

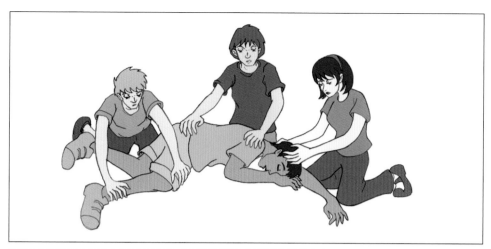

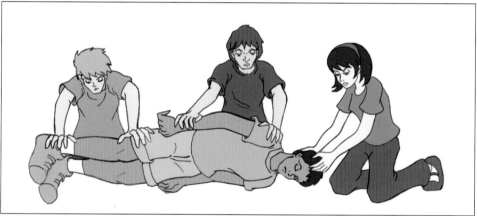

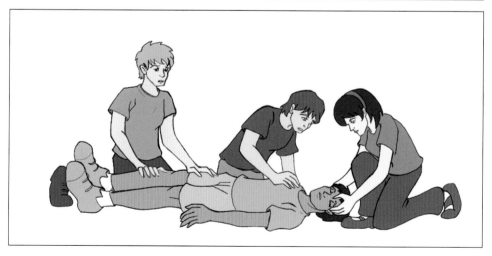

Two-person log roll.

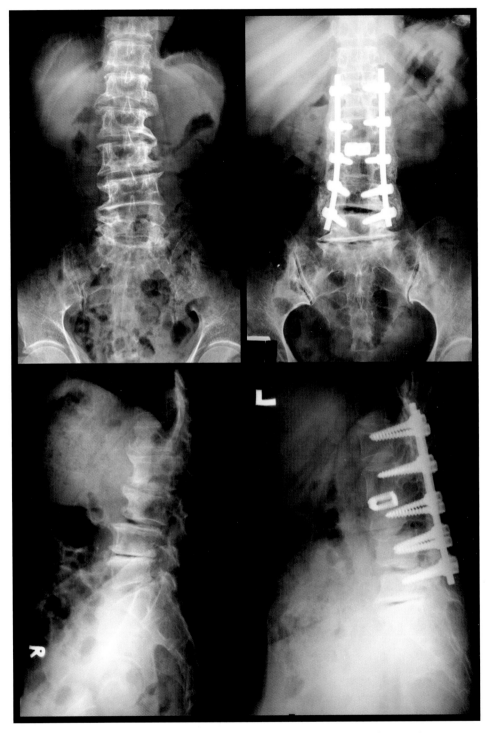

In the event of a spinal injury, evacuation is necessary so that a doctor can determine the source of the injury that may require surgical fixation.

Focused Assessment of Cervical Spine (FACS)

(Only perform if trained and comfortable with this procedure.)
- The patient is sober, alert, and cooperative.
- No strength deficits in hand grip, wiggling of fingers, and foot–push/pull.
- No sensation deficits in upper or lower limbs (sharp vs dull differentiation).
- No painful injury that may distract the patient from the presence of neck pain.
- No tenderness to pushing on the upper (neck) midline bony prominences.

Check your FACS

If patient is alert, sober, has no point tenderness to midline neck vertebrae, has no sensation or motor deficits, and has no distracting painful injuries, *and* can rotate head 45 degrees to either shoulder, and touch chin to chest without pain in the middle of the neck (side of neck pain is okay, as this is likely from sore neck muscles), you can "clear" the upper spine without concern for a serious spinal injury or need for further neck immobilization.

Treatment

- Stabilize the spine by manually holding the head "in-line" with the rest of the body.
- Apply neck immobilization (e.g., molded SAM splint, backpack waist belt, etc.).
- Any log roll or movement done in small increments.
- If a litter is needed (*see* **Appendix B**), ensure to apply maximum padding around bony points and under knees and lower back with awareness of protection from the environment (e.g., cold, wet, sun, etc.) and removal of wet clothing.

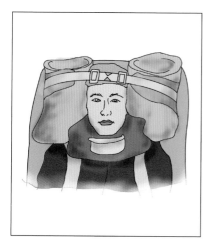
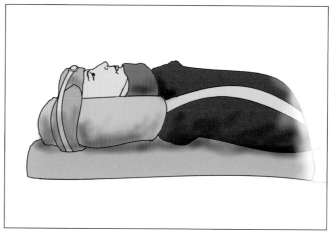

Improvised cervical spine immobilization.

Evacuate: Any patient who has a possible spinal injury (cannot be cleared by FACS or cannot walk due to pain).

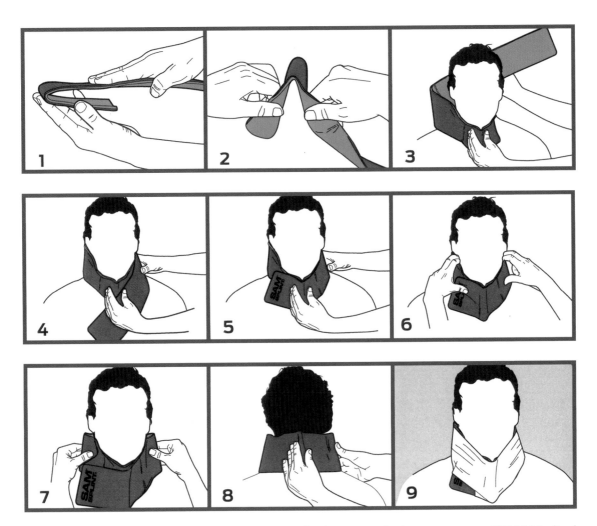

SAM splint molded cervical collar. *Images and splinting technique courtesy of SAM Medical.*

SCOUTING GUIDE TO WILDERNESS FIRST AID

CHAPTER 28

WOUND CARE

Most bleeding is obvious with a quick visual inspection. Blood from low pressure veins flowing out, and blood from arteries spurting out with the pumping heart, can be life-threatening. Controlling the bleeding may be the first step in the resuscitative care of an injured person. During the secondary assessment, be sure to check under a person's clothes with a hand sweep and look underneath them, to ensure there are no places of disguised blood loss.

Serious blood loss can occur internally from an injured organ or bleeding vessel that may not be visible or obvious. Always consider the MOI of the injury, and be aware of symptoms of progressive blood loss (e.g., dizziness exacerbated with sitting up or standing, rapid pulse, fatigue and weakness on exertion, and worsening pain and/or tenderness of the abdomen or other part of the body).

Wound management in the backcountry involves three steps: (1) control bleeding, (2) irrigation, and (3) wound closure. Always use gloves and universal

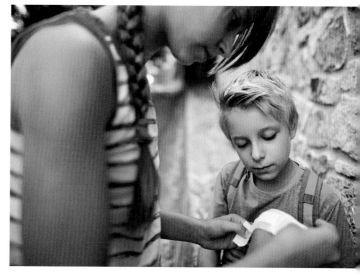

Wound care is essential in the backcountry—even a small cut can get infected.

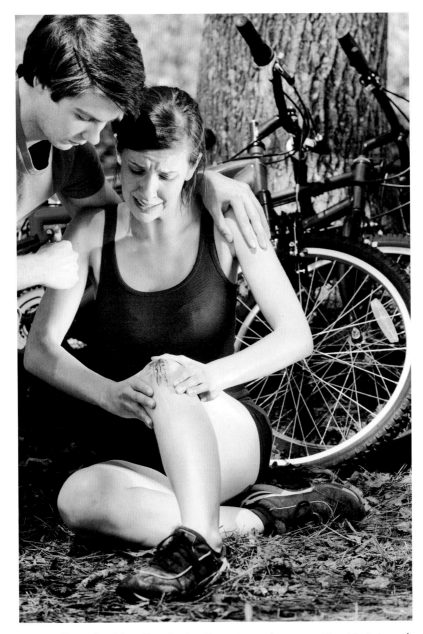

Controlling the bleeding is the first step when a patient is injured.

precautions when dealing with body fluids to avoid transmission of blood borne diseases. Most wounds are simple and will stop with direct pressure and elevation—very rarely are tourniquets indicated. Remember that any tourniquet may lead to eventual limb amputation,

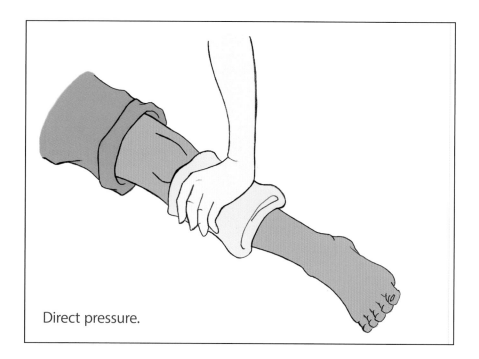

Direct pressure.

so use only as a last resort when life-threatening bleeding is occurring—when it's "Life or Limb." Any wound that occurs in the backcountry is at risk of getting infected. Copious irrigation and flushing out all visible foreign matter is the first step to minimizing poor outcomes. Any water that is safe to drink is safe to flush a wound with. Finally, closing a wound may optimize aesthetic outcome but increases the risk of infection. Wounds that are not closed should be packed with clean/sterile gauze and allowed to drain and heal on their own.

Treatment: Controlling Bleeding

- Direct pressure (on a small surface area, using a clean gauze bandage) for ten to fifteen minutes. Can use compressive wrap. The smaller the area of the compressive dressing directly on the wound, the greater the pressure exerted.
- If possible, elevate extremity above level of heart.
- Can apply a moist regular tea bag to wound to assist with bleeding control.
- If the patient has continued extremity bleeding despite the aforementioned methods, and there is concern that they may bleed to death, consider a tourniquet—"Life or Limb!"

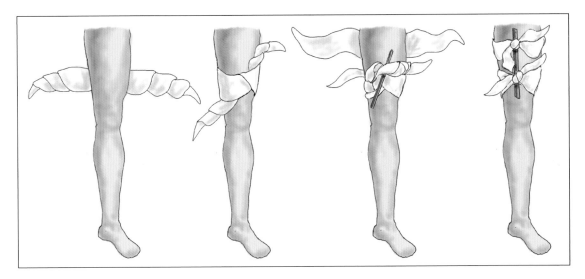

Tourniquet.

Tourniquet

1. Secure a band of cloth (at least two inches wide) two inches above extremity wound (between wound and the heart), as close to the lowest joint as possible. Do not place over the joint.
2. Tie half an overhand knot, put a small stick or rod on top of knot, and finish the half overhand knot over it The stick is the windlass that will tighten the tourniquet and provide mechanical advantage..
3. Tighten tourniquet by turning stick until bleeding stops. Secure the stick (tape or another cloth knot).
4. Loosen the tourniquet in twenty minutes to check for bleeding. If bleeding continues, reapply tourniquet and note time of application.
   If bleeding has stopped, leave tourniquet off.

Remember: Applying a tourniquet may result in limb amputation.

Treatment: Irrigation

- Irrigate the wound with forceful pressure with an irrigation syringe, drinking tube from a hydration bladder or sports bottle, or poke a hole (diameter

If water is safe to drink, then it is safe to irrigate a wound with.

  SCOUTING GUIDE TO WILDERNESS FIRST AID

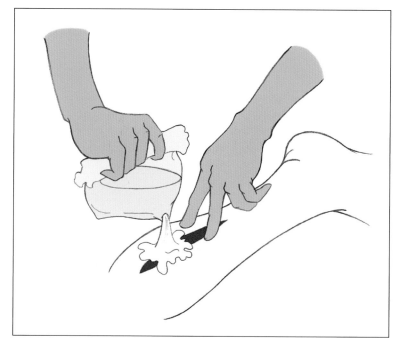

Wound irrigation.

of one safety pin) in the corner of a plastic bag, squeezing water out onto wound, using at least one liter of drinkable water.

- Pull wound edges apart for thorough cleaning.
- Abrasions should be scrubbed with soap and water.
- Any water safe to drink is safe to irrigate with.

Treatment: Wound Closure

- Wounds with edges that can be approximated may be closed: Use wound closure strips or paper tape to tape the wound shut. Apply tape perpendicular to wound, opposing the edges. Apply another piece of tape and/or benzoin adhesive perpendicular to anchor the strips.
- Cover with antibiotic ointment and gauze dressing.
- Change dressing every twenty-four hours.

Use gauze to cover the wound, and be sure to change the dressing every twenty-four hours.

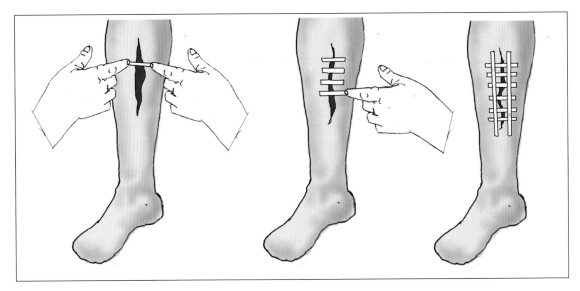

Wound closure.

- **Do Not Close:** puncture wounds, animal bites, or heavily contaminated wounds.
- Gaping or poorly opposed wounds may be left open to minimize infection. Apply antibiotic ointment (Bacitracin), cover with sterile/clean nonstick gauze, cover with gauze/wrap dressing.
- If wound is on joint of extremity, consider splinting wound.

⚠ **Red Flags:** Signs of infection, including pus, redness, streaking.

Treatment: Scalp Lacerations

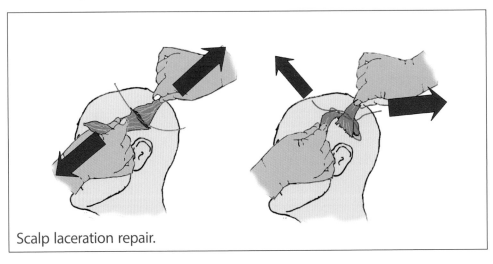

Scalp laceration repair.

- Take a strand of thread, fishing line, or thin string and lay it on top of (parallel to) the wound.
- Take strands of long hair on either side of the laceration and then cross them over, bringing the opposing wound edges together.
- Have another person tie a square knot with the thread as you hold the wound closed with hair.
- Repeat as many times as necessary down the length of the wound until the laceration is closed.

Treatment: Impaled Object

- Do not remove a large impaled object, as the object may be compressing and plugging shut injured tissues and its removal may lead to severe bleeding.
- Put a bulky dressing around the object to stabilize it.
- Secure the dressing well.
- Evacuate.

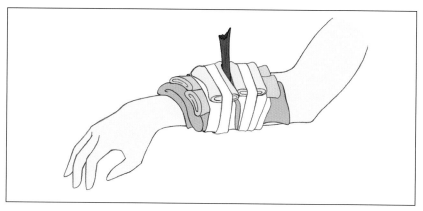

Impaled object.

Treatment: Embedded Fishhook

- Tie a string or shoelace around the bend of the hook.
- Push the shaft of the fishhook toward the barb/skin surface (this disengages the barb).
- Pull the string up and away at a 30-degree angle, yanking the hook from the skin with a snapping motion.

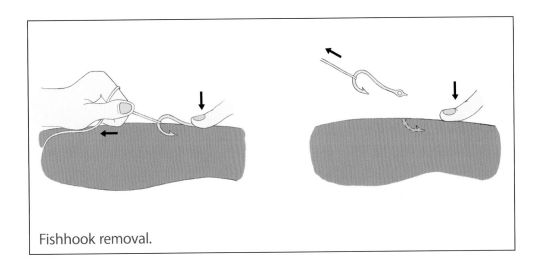

Fishhook removal.

🚁 **Evacuate:**

- Any amputation, tourniquet usage, or impaled object.
- Any wound that is heavily contaminated, is from a bite (human or animal), involves a joint space, or which may involve underlying tendons or ligaments (loss of range of motion of hand, foot, finger, or toe).
- Any wound infection.
- Any concern for hidden injury/internal bleeding.

SCOUTING GUIDE TO WILDERNESS FIRST AID

APPENDIX A
MEDICATION INFORMATION

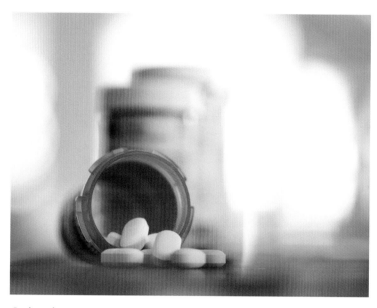

Only take prescription medication if you have been instructed by a physician or if someone's life is in danger without that medicine.

Do not provide prescription medicine unless you are a physician, have been instructed by a physician, or feel that someone's life is in danger if you do not give the medicine. Always ask about allergies prior to dispensing any *medicine.*

In addition to having medication administration protocols, you should obtain informed consent for medication administration, even nonprescription medication. Inform the

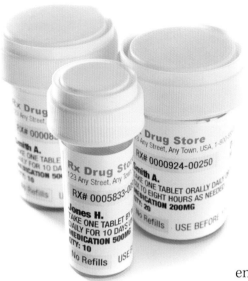

recipient of the indications, contraindications, and possible side effects of the medication, and obtain consent to administer. Before administering any medication, read the protocols, confirm the dosage, read the label to confirm the medication, ask the patient about previous history with this medication and any known allergies, and ask the patient if he or she is currently on any other medications and, if so, review the protocols for contraindications.

All dosing is indicated for adults. Listed medicines as generic names as well as commonly encountered brand names.

Before administering medication, be sure to read the label for instructions and dosage.

Abbreviations

PO   Oral
IM   Intramuscular injection
OTC   Over-the-counter
Rx   Prescription

Medication Quick Guide

Pain Relief OTC

Acetaminophen   *(Tylenol)*
Ibuprofen   *(Advil, Motrin)*
Naproxen   *(Aleve)*

Anti-Allergy OTC

Hydrocortisone cream
Diphenhydramine   *(Benadryl)*
Famotidine   *(Pepcid)*

Anti-Allergy Rx
Albuterol
Epinephrine   *(EpiPen)*

Antibiotic OTC
Polymyxin/bacitracin   *(Polysporin)*

Anti-Diarrheal OTC
Loperamide hydrochloride *(Imodium)*
Bismuth subsalicylate   *(Pepto-Bismol)*

Anti-Nausea OTC
Famotidine   *(Pepcid)*
Bismuth subsalicylate   *(Pepto-Bismol)*

Pain Relief OTC

Acetaminophen (Tylenol)

Classification: Non-narcotic pain relief, anti-fever.

Dose: See directions on label.

Indications: For relief of pain due to headache, cold, and flu discomfort, minor muscle and joint discomfort, and menstrual cramps. For reduction of fever. Especially useful for those allergic to aspirin or ibuprofen. Does not control inflammation.

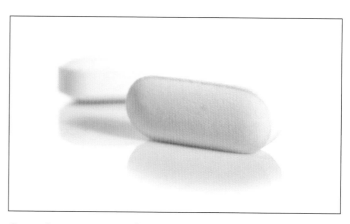

Generic acetaminophen.

Contraindications: Hypersensitivity, active alcoholism, liver disease, hepatitis. Acetaminophen is a common ingredient in over-the-counter pain, cold, and flu medicine. Be careful of accidental overdose in combination with other products.

Side Effects: Hypersensitivity rare.

Ibuprofen (Advil, Motrin)
Classification: Non-narcotic pain relief, anti-fever, non-steroidal anti-inflammatory.
Dose: See directions on label.
Indications: For symptomatic relief of pain associated with headache, colds, flu, frostbite, toothache, arthritis, burns, and menstrual cramps. May be used to reduce fever. For pain of inflammation and reduction of inflammation associated with muscle, joint, and over-use injuries. For prevention of acute mountain sickness and treatment of high altitude headache.
Contraindications: Active stomach or intestinal ulcer, gastrointestinal bleeding disorder, history of hypersensitivity to aspirin or other non-steroidal anti-inflammatory drugs.
Side Effects: Nausea, abdominal pain, dizziness, rash.

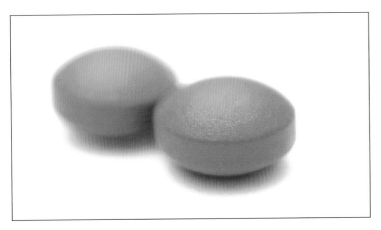

Generic ibuprofen.

Naproxen (Aleve)
Classification: Non-narcotic pain relief, anti-fever, non-steroidal anti-inflammatory.
Dose: See directions on label.
Indications: For relief of pain from headache, tooth-ache, arthritis, muscle aches, tendinitis, and menstrual cramps. May be used to reduce fever and to

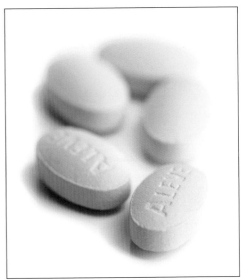

Aleve.

  SCOUTING GUIDE TO WILDERNESS FIRST AID

treat pain of inflammation and reduction of inflammation associated with muscle, joint, and over-use injuries.

Contraindications: Active stomach or intestinal ulcer, gastrointestinal bleeding disorder, history of hypersensitivity to aspirin or other non-steroidal anti-inflammatory drugs.

Side Effects: Nausea, upset stomach, heartburn, headache, dizziness, drowsiness, bruising, and rash.

Anti-Allergy OTC

Hydrocortisone cream

Classification: Glucocorticoid (steroid)

Dose: See directions on label.

Indications: For relief of pain and itching of jellyfish stings, poison ivy, oak, stinging nettles, sumac, insect bites, and other allergic skin reactions. May help dry up oozing rash of allergic skin reactions.

Contraindications: Infections.

Side Effects: Itching, redness, irritation

Diphenhydramine (Benadryl)

Classification: Antihistamine (H1-blocker)

Dose: For adults, 25–50mg/6 hours PO

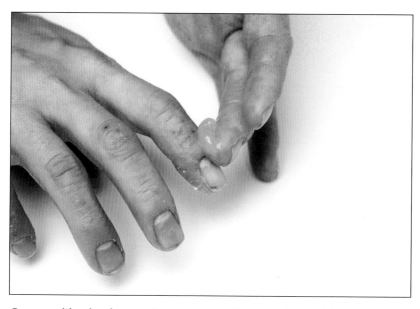

Creams like hydrocortisone can relieve pain and itching from allergic skin reactions.

Indications: For temporary relief of respiratory allergy symptoms and cold symptoms. Helps relieve the itching of allergic skin reactions. Useful in treatment of mild, moderate, and severe allergic and anaphylactic reactions. May be used as a mild sedative and for insomnia. May help alleviate seasickness.

Contraindications: Hypersensitivity, acute asthma attack, glaucoma, peptic ulcer.

Side Effects: Drowsiness, dizziness, weakness, dry mouth, thickening lung secretions, inability to urinate.

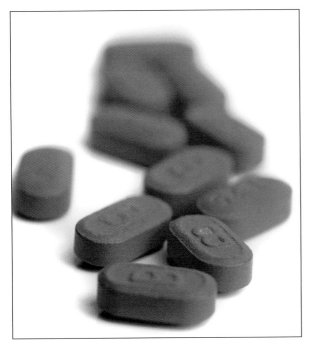

Benadryl.

Famotidine (Pepcid)

Classification: Antihistamine (H2-blocker)

Dose: See directions on label.

Indications: For heartburn, acid stomach, and ulcer disease. Useful in treatment of "sour stomach," and moderate and severe allergic and anaphylactic reactions.

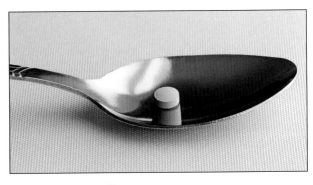

A famotidine pill.

Contraindications: Hypersensitivity to famotidine or other H2-blockers.

Side Effects: Constipation, diarrhea, dizziness, headache.

Anti-Allergy Rx

Albuterol

Classification: Bronchodilator

Dose: See directions on label.

Indications: Shortness of breath or breathing difficulty thought to be secondary to reactive airway disease (asthma) or anaphylaxis.

Contraindications: Fast heart rate secondary to underlying heart condition.

Side Effects: Palpitations, fast heart rate, tremor.

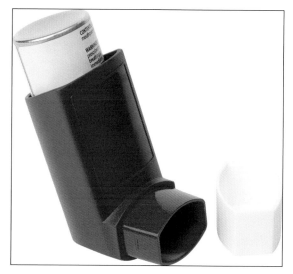

Albuterol can be administered through an inhaler.

Epinephrine (EpiPen)

Classification: Bronchodilator, antiallergenic, cardiac stimulant.

Dose: See directions on label.

Indications: For severe allergic reactions including anaphylaxis and severe asthma attack.

Contraindications: No true contraindications with anaphylaxis, hypertension, cardiac disease, glaucoma, shock.

Side Effects: Increased heart rate, nervousness, dizziness, lightheadedness, nausea, headache.

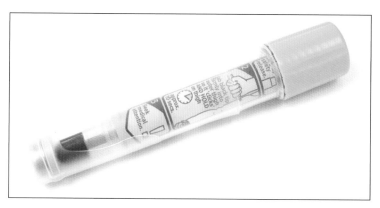

Follow directions to correctly and safely dispense epinephrine, often from an EpiPen.

Antibiotic OTC

Polymyxin B sulfate/bacitracin (Polysporin)

Classification: Antibiotic

Dose: See directions on label.

Indications: Contains ingredients for prevention of infection in minor wounds. Works as a lubricant, offers some relief from itching.

Contraindications: Hypersensitivity.

Side Effects: Hypersensitivity reactions: burning, itching, inflammation, contact dermatitis.

Anti-Diarrheal OTC

Loperamide hydrochloride (Imodium)

Classification: Antidiarrheal

Dose: See directions on label.

Indications: For use in the control of diarrhea. Thought to limit peristalsis. Helpful in evacuating someone with severe diarrhea.

Contraindications: Hypersensitivity, bloody stool.

Side Effects: Dry mouth, dizziness, abdominal discomfort.

Bismuth subsalicylate (Pepto-Bismol)

Classification: Antidiarrheal

Dose: See directions on label.

Indications: For use in the control of diarrhea.

Contraindications: Hypersensitivity to aspirin.

Side Effects: Gray-black stool/tongue, nausea/vomiting, constipation, ringing in ears.

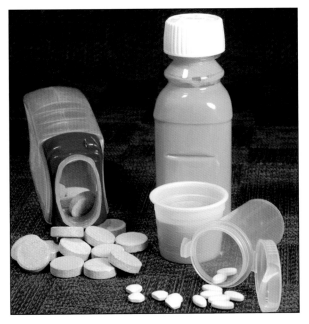

Pepto-Bismol comes in both liquid and tablet form.

Anti-Nausea OTC

Bismuth subsalicylate (Pepto-Bismol) chewable tablets

Classification: Anti-diarrheal.

Dose: See directions on label.

Indications: For use in the control of nausea.

Contraindications: Hypersensitivity to aspirin.

Side Effects: Gray-black stool/tongue, nausea/vomiting, constipation, ringing in ears.

Famotidine (Pepcid)

Classification: Antihistamine (H2-blocker).

Dose: See directions on label.

Indications: For heartburn, "sour stomach," and ulcer disease. Can be used in conjunction with Phenergan for nausea. Useful in treatment of moderate allergic and anaphylactic reactions.

Contraindications: Hypersensitivity to famotidine or other H2-blockers.

Side Effects: Constipation, diarrhea, dizziness, headache.

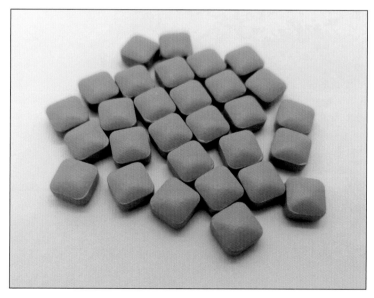

Another kind of famotidine pill.

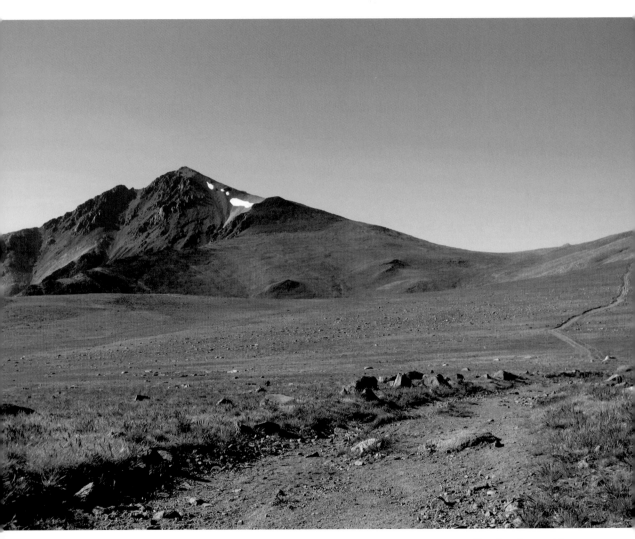

APPENDIX B
EVACUATION INFORMATION

One of the most difficult decisions in wilderness medicine is whether to evacuate a victim. Not only is an evacuation prematurely ending an adventure, but as there is often substantial money, time, and training that went into the trip planning, there are multiple variables at risk of being lost. But safety needs to be the top priority. Be aware of the "red flags" for the disease process in play, and early preparation and planning will be an advantage before issues progress. It is preferable to assist someone during the day than to extricate them with a stretcher at night! A potential evacuation is an undertaking with multiple hazards that need to be taken into account prior to embarking: changing environmental conditions, maneuvering an injured person over inclement terrain, worsening of the victim's condition, and support for and needs of the rescuers.

Evacuation Tips

- Remember to have shelter. Evacuations take longer than expected, so prepare for an overnight bivouac or unexpected weather. As a French mountain guide once told me in the Karakorum, "You could die up there. Bring a tent."
- If you send a messenger to get help, write down the salient medical and logistical information so the rescuers can both locate and bring appropriate resources.
- It is next to impossible to carry any but the lightest victim over any substantial distances. For example, it takes six to eight trained rescuers to extricate an adult. While

the concept of a litter system or rope carry is attractive, exhausting the rescuers from futile attempts will not benefit anyone.

- If using an improvised stretcher, make it as comfortable as possible—you cannot use enough padding.
- Remember empathy. There are limited resources available in the wilderness first-aid kit to treat the hurt and fear of the victim. Often the most useful tools are reassurance, commiseration, and empathy. The rescuer suddenly has the responsibility of a dependent who may be incapacitated, and it is reasonable to assign an individual in the rescue party to look out for the victim's needs (e.g. hunger, thirst, toilet, and comfort, etc.).

Daisy Chain Litter System

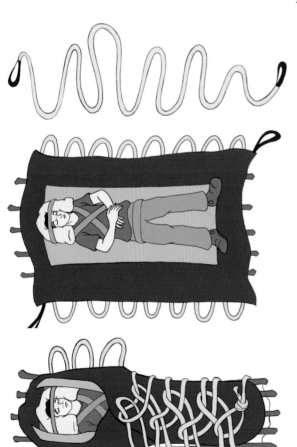

Daisy chain litter.

Materials needed:

- Rope, at least eighty feet (twenty-five meters) long.
- Tarp or tent fly.
- Sleeping bag or sleeping pad.

Instructions:

1. Lay out the daisy chain; loops are arms' width (six feet), with fifteen to twenty loops.

2. Lay tarp and/or padding on the rope and package the patient.

3. Tie a loop knot with a bight (figure 8) at the foot end of the rope. Wrap the patient, cinching and looping each successive length towards the head, then tie off the rope.

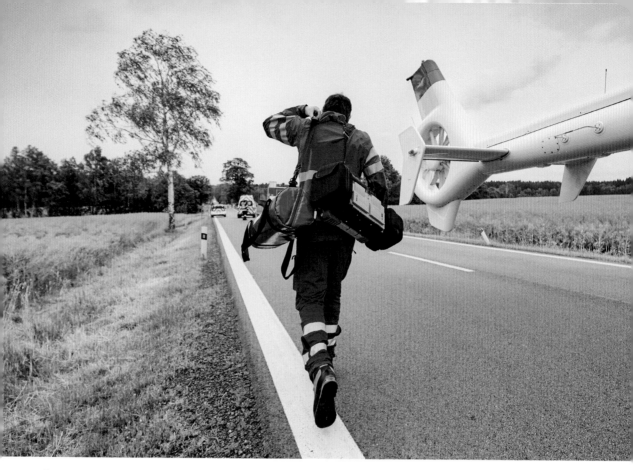

If a patient has a better chance of recovery with an air evacuation, a helicopter evacuation can be considered.

Helicopter Rescue and Safety

Conditions for Helicopter Evacuation

- The victim's chances of recovery are better with air than they are with ground evacuation.
- A ground evacuation would be arduous or unduly dangerous to either victim or the rescuers.
- The helicopter pilot and crew would be functioning within their safety protocols.

Information for Helicopter Team

- Number of patients.
- Patients' weight and medical status.

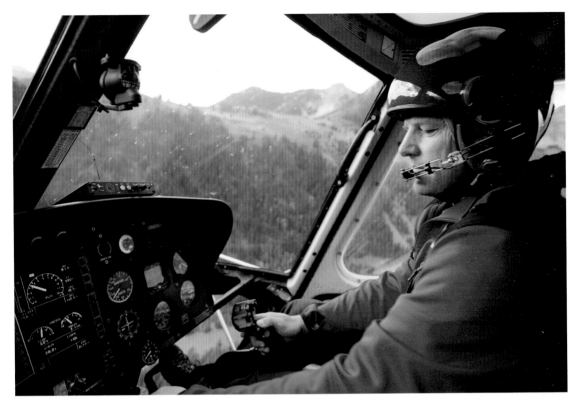

The helicopter pilot must operate within their safety protocols during an evacuation.

- Wind direction at landing zone.
- Weather conditions at landing zone.
- UTM or latitude/longitude coordinates and altitude.
- Geographical description of landing zone.

Do-Not-Fly Conditions
- Winds over 40 mph (70 Km/hr).
- Night flight into mountainous areas.
- Low visibility.
- Poor or unknown landing conditions.
- Slopes of more than 10 degrees.

Safety Rules
- Never approach a helicopter until signaled to do so by the pilot or crew.
- Keep in line-of-sight view of the pilot and crew.

  SCOUTING GUIDE TO WILDERNESS FIRST AID

- Clear away debris prior to helicopter approach, then stay clear of the landing zone.
- Stand outside landing zone with back to the wind, facing the approach.
- Approach from downhill.
- *Do not* approach from uphill.
- Avoid the tail rotor.

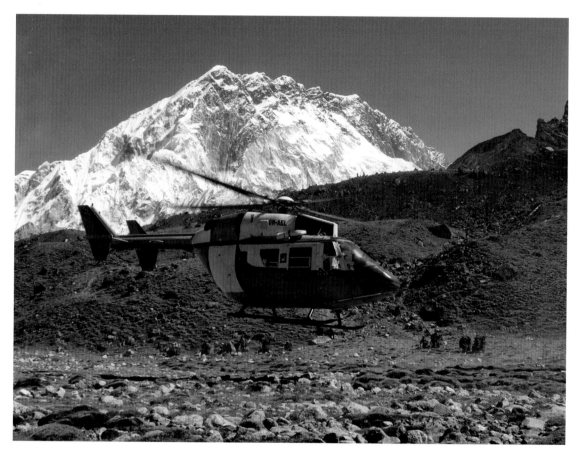

Move outside the landing zone when the helicopter approaches. *Credit: Grant Lipman*

Landing Zone Set-Up

- Day: 100 feet x 100 feet (thirty big paces).
- Night: 150 feet x 150 feet (fifty big paces).
- Mark location/corners of landing zone with brightly colored objects/clothes that can show wind direction.

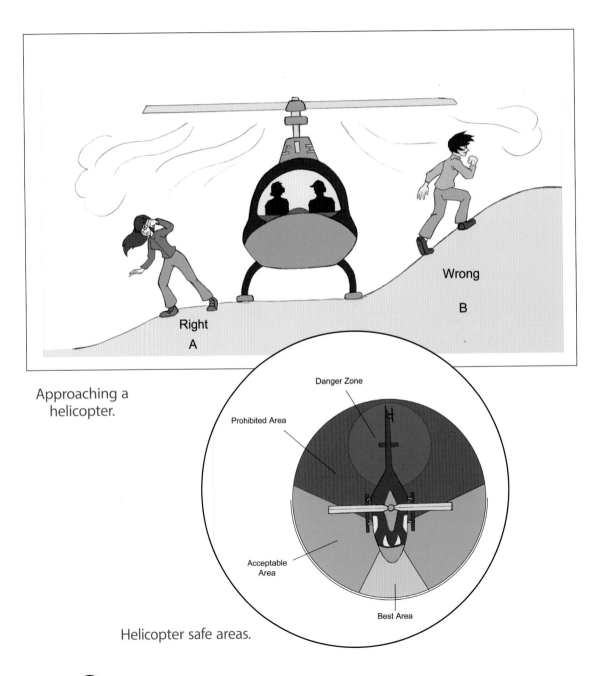

Approaching a
helicopter.

Right
A

Wrong

B

Danger Zone

Prohibited Area

Acceptable
Area

Best Area

Helicopter safe areas.

SCOUTING GUIDE TO WILDERNESS FIRST AID

APPENDIX C
FIRST AID KIT

Basic First-Aid Kit

√   SAM splint
√   Scissors
√   Safety pins
√   Duct tape
√   Wound closure strips (1/4" x 4")
√   Benzoin (liquid adhesive) prep pads
√   Alcohol prep pads
√   Elastikon (3")
√   Paper tape
√   Spenco 2nd Skin (1" pads)
√   Latex or nitrile gloves
√   CPR microshield mask
√   Cotton swabs
√   4" x 4" gauze dressing
√   Compression bandage wrap
√   Sunblock

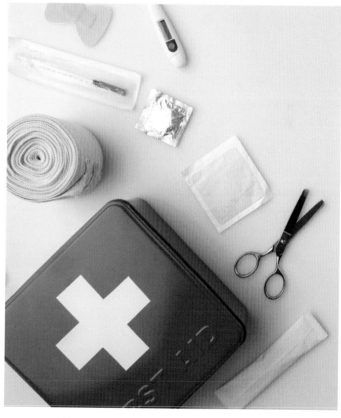

Bring a first-aid kid when you travel into the wilderness.

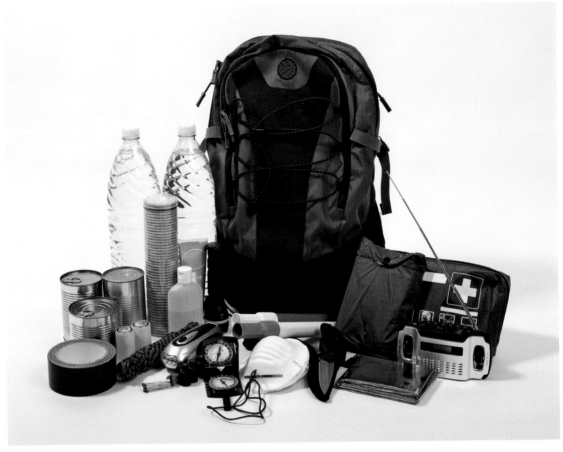

Prepare all of your survival essentials before going on a wilderness outing.

Survival Essentials

√ Emergency space blanket
√ Whistle
√ Water bottle and water purification system
√ Food
√ Headlamp and batteries
√ Map/compass/GPS
√ Fire starter system
√ Signal mirror
√ Appropriate clothes/rain shell
√ Parachute cord (4 mm or 3/16")—fifty feet